The Beautiful Journey

The Beautiful Journey

Finding Purpose Through Cancer

ANDREA DYAN CAMPBELL

DANNIE BOY PUBLISHING
CLEVELAND

The Beautiful Journey: Finding Purpose Through Cancer

Copyright © 2016 Andrea Dyan Campbell

Exterior design by Rhonda "Turquoiz" White

Cover and back photography by Terri Moorefield
www.TerriMoorefieldPhotography.com

Library of Congress Control Number: 2016912811

ISBN 978-0-9966208-1-9

Contents

Dedication

This book is dedicated to my biggest supporter
and champion, my first love, my mom, Jeri
Campbell; my dad, Dannie Baker, who
recently ascended to heaven; and to my
99.9-year-old grandmother Katie, whom I
affectionately call Woman.

Also...

To those who battled cancer and are no longer with us,
you are not forgotten: my sister Crystal Olivia McCad-
den; my brother, Danny Baker; my aunt Paula Campbell; my coach, mentor and dear friend, Sharon Piper-
Diggs. You are deeply missed and will always hold a
special place in my heart.

To all the survivors and those who are currently in the
fight, know that you are not alone. I stand with you.

Here's My Why...

"Everybody should have to have cancer!" I know that sounds crazy, but please let me explain. Cancer is a yucky, ugly, horrible disease that I wish would go away forever. I wouldn't wish it on anyone. However, I do wish that everyone could experience my beautiful transformation that occurred as a result of my battle with cancer. I am not the same person I was before. I am stronger, wiser, braver, more faithful, more appreciative, more mature, more giving, more resilient, more beautiful, and just plain ole more. I truly admire and respect the person I've become. Also, as a result of my battle, my relationship with God is much stronger and deeper than it's ever been.

After my diagnosis with breast cancer, a friend suggested that I chronicle my journey through cancer in a blog. This book, *The Beautiful Journey*, is based on those blogs. All the emotions that you'll read are my raw, honest feelings. You'll experience all the ups and downs, the good and the bad. You will see how my faith in God helped me claim victory over cancer. Also, you'll see how going through this adversity led me to my purpose.

As a survivor, I believe it is my responsibility to share my experiences and show how God is still in the miracle business. Yes, it may have taken me a while to actually put pen to paper, but as Anna Wintour said, "It's always about timing. If it's too soon, no one understands. If it's too late, everyone's forgotten." I believe that last year was too soon. I was still living out my story and I needed to get to a place where I felt comfortable revisiting that part of my life. Now is the time. I am finally ready to share my story...before people forget. Before I forget.

Even though I would rather not think about all that I had to go through during that time, I can't escape it. This was my life. My joint pains and many scars (which I consider my battle wounds) serve as a reminder of all that I had to overcome to become victorious.

My intention for sharing my story isn't to make you feel sorry for me or my situation. Instead, I want to inspire you as you go through your own trials and tribulations, whether it happens to be cancer, some other ailment or even a stronghold that has you bound. After the blog entries, I've included my personal reflections of those moments years later.

Also, at the end of each chapter, there are some questions for you to reflect on. I wanted to create the opportunity for you to insert yourself in the book and go on your own personal beautiful journey. Regardless of the situation, the common thread for victory is believing and trusting in God's word. His word tells us that all things work together for good. Even in the darkest storm, God is still in control.

I am stepping outside of my comfort zone and allowing God to use me through the talents He has graciously given me. I am appreciative of this opportunity and platform to share my story. If I can just encourage one person to hold on and trust God, and to check their breasts regularly, this book will not be in vain. I just want to help save a life or a soul.

Thank you for taking the time to follow my beautiful journey.

Foreword

When I first met Andrea, or Dreaaaaa, as I often call her, I recognized the light she exuded. We were at a work event and although I'd spent months in preparation for this very important event where I'd be speaking to over 2,000 healthcare specialists, Drea's light caused me to lose focus.

Let me explain, I prepare for each and every speaking event right up to the moment of delivery. I speak to millions of people every year and when I do, I prepare my head and my heart to connect to everyone in the room. I don't hang out the night before or chummy up to the big wigs afterwards.

I'm there for everyone. So when Drea's glow distracted me from my notes, just minutes before my event, I knew that she was one of those folks my mother would have called an old soul; someone who is young in years, but has something we all need to know.

We chatted a little before the event and I felt compelled to share my direct contact information.

It took her a while to connect. When she did, I didn't ask why, I listened.

As I did, I heard the heart of one who'd been on a journey; several in fact. Upon her return, she had something to share.

Drea and I began to do what I call Sherapy Sessions; a type of therapy I developed with my friend Brynn Grant. In these structured and yet free flowing sessions, we connect and heal through the sharing of stories.

When we discussed goals and dreams, Drea told me that she was working on a book about her journey. As she spoke of the pain and hardship, all I could hear was her smile. I saw her bright eyes and willing heart and I heard one who gave and gave in the midst of her own pain. I saw her light.

"You should call this the Beautiful Journey," I said.

Drea laughed, music oozing from the joy of that laughter. "Beautiful?" She managed in disbelief.

And then I shared my own truth. I told her that for all of the weeks that we'd been sharing stories of loss and pain and learning, she had been helping me.

Our weekly Sherapy sessions helped me to reframe my own head injury, foot surgery, battle with adult onset asthma, and loss of loved ones. As we walked through Drea's recovery, I was recovering as well.

Her journey to wellness was my journey to beautiful.

I told Drea that through her pain she had become incredibly beautiful.

She stopped laughing and said something that only an analytical person can say, "I'll think about it."

Now I laughed, because I knew that the teacher had become the student and my wonderful time with Drea was coming to an end.

The Beautiful Journey is not another one of those books about some isolated incident for someone you may or may not know. It is not about cancer, illness or loss; it is about transformation.

It's about finding yourself through your struggle/ life and reclaiming the abundant joy you were always meant to have.

In to each life, a little rain must fall. When it does, may you also become your beautiful true self.

Bertice Berry, PhD.

1

my story

THEREFORE DO NOT WORRY ABOUT TOMORROW,
FOR TOMORROW WILL WORRY ABOUT ITSELF. EACH
DAY HAS ENOUGH TROUBLE OF ITS OWN.

– MATTHEW 6:34

———————

Thursday, October 8, 2009 was officially the worst day of my life. Besides it being the birthday of my deceased sister, Crystal, it was also the day I received the worst news.

"YOU HAVE CANCER."

Wait, did I hear her correctly? What was I supposed to say to that? I was completely caught off guard and stunned. While trying to process what I just heard, all these emotions came over me. This wasn't the news I expected to hear, and of course it was not the news I wanted to hear. My heart was physically aching.

There I was, sitting in a patient's room at Cleveland Clinic, a world renowned hospital. I was visiting my childhood friend, Cassandra, who was recuperating from a complication due to a previous operation. Just the night before, she had to have emergency surgery and barely escaped death.

As we sat there talking about everything that had taken place with her health crisis, my cell phone rang. I looked at it and noticed that it was a call from my doctor's office. Although I was expecting a call to discuss the results of my breast biopsy, I thought it wouldn't be for another of couple of days. Anxiously and somewhat nervously, I answered the call.

"Hello?"

On the other end of the line, I heard a voice say, "Andrea?"

I replied, "Yes, this is she."

After confirming that it was indeed me on the telephone, my doctor begrudgingly told me the results. "I am so sorry to have to tell you this, but your biopsy came back positive."

Is she saying that I...wait, what? I was shocked and confused.

"Huh? What are you saying? Are you saying I have cancer?"

Those words didn't even sound right coming out of my mouth. I was hoping my ears were playing tricks on me. Perhaps I didn't hear what I thought I did. Yes, that's it. I misunderstood what she said.

She answered, "Yes, you have breast cancer. I am very sorry to have to give you bad news, but I wanted to let you know as soon as possible."

In that moment, I was scared to death. Scared *of* death. I felt sad and unsure about what my future held. Tears began to roll down my face.

Cassandra noticed how distraught I was and she tried to console me. In her haste to comfort me, she yanked off her EKG patches and somehow managed to get out of her bed and walk over to me. She began rubbing my back and continuously asked me what was going on. I hadn't told her that I had a biopsy performed on my right breast.

I couldn't even form the words to tell her what the doctor said because I was crying so hard. Eventually I was finally able to mumble, "*I...have...breast cancer.*" I'm not even sure how she was able to understand what I was saying underneath all the sobbing.

She kept rubbing my back and telling me that everything would be alright. Some seconds later, a nurse came rushing into the room. She was in a panic. She thought my girlfriend had died because the EKG monitors showed that her heart had flatlined.

Once the nurse saw that my girlfriend was alive, she asked what was going on. Cassandra told her that I had just found out I had breast cancer. The nurse walked over to me and brought me some tissue. As I wiped my tears and cleaned my runny nose, she reached out her arms, pulled me in toward her and gave me a tight hug.

Afterward, she grabbed my hands, looked me in my eyes, and calmly said, "I know that it's difficult being diagnosed with cancer, but that just means you now have the responsibility of being a survivor."

What was she saying? I have the responsibility of being a survivor? I looked her dead in her eyes and asked her what she meant by that.

She said, "Being diagnosed doesn't necessarily mean death. Now, you have the responsibility to fight your hardest to win this battle. And once you do, you can help others do the same."

Her words struck a chord with me. I looked at

her and thought, *You're right.* In that moment, she brought joy inside my tears. My entire perspective changed about my diagnosis. I wiped my tears and accepted my new responsibility...to be a survivor.

Now, the words, *"You have breast cancer,"* didn't have the same effect on me. Being diagnosed with breast cancer did not necessarily mean I would be defeated. I could be victorious. I *would* be victorious!

Unfortunately, I do not know the name of the nurse who came into the room that day, but I am forever indebted to her. She changed my life. At that moment, her words gave me hope, and I welcomed my new role...a survivor.

Even though I was somewhat feeling better about my situation, the worst part wasn't over. I still had to tell my mom about my diagnosis. How was I going to muster up the courage to tell her that I had breast cancer?

Just like Cassandra, my mother wasn't aware that I had a biopsy. I didn't think there was a need to worry her about *nothing*, since that's exactly what I thought it was...*nothing*.

For the past few months, I'd been experiencing sharp, stabbing pains in my right breast. I decided I would try to figure out what was going on with me. I searched the Internet for "pain in breast" and had pretty much figured out what was wrong *...so I thought.* After my self-diagnosis of fibroadenoma, I confidently went into my biopsy knowing that was what was causing the constant shooting pains. Never did I think it could be breast cancer. That thought didn't even cross my mind until the biopsy was performed.

During the biopsy, the doctor mentioned that she wasn't sure what the mass was.

"It could be cancer, but I won't know until I receive the results from the biopsy."

That was when I began to second guess my self-diagnosis. When she said that it *could be cancer*, it really hit me. Could this really be something much more than what I thought, something much more serious?

Although the doctor's tone was calm when she said that she wasn't sure if the mass was cancer, the rest of her conversation, her actions, and the actions of the nursing staff pretty much told a different story. The nurse who assisted with the biopsy was rubbing my back, holding my hand, and telling me, "If it is breast cancer, it's curable." She also gave me a hug as I left procedure room.

I was confused and scared. Of course a few tears ran down my face, but I kept telling myself that everything would be alright. There was still hope that the results were going to come back negative. Right?

Well, looking back, I know that wasn't the case. Unfortunately, I was diagnosed with breast cancer at the age of 39. After I received that phone call, my thoughts were, *Now what? Where do I go from here?* One minute I'm enjoying life and then the next, I'm having to face death. You have to be kidding me.

My life changed that quickly, in the blink of an eye.

―――――――――

Reflection Questions

1. *What were the circumstances where your life changed in an instant?*
2. *What was your reaction?*
3. *Who did you tell?*
4. *What was your new responsibility?*

2

plans interrupted

"GOD WILL NOT PERMIT ANY TROUBLES TO COME
UPON US, UNLESS HE HAS A SPECIFIC PLAN BY WHICH
GREAT BLESSING CAN COME OUT OF THE DIFFICULTY."

— PETER MARSHALL

Having breast cancer was surreal. As you can imagine, this was a lot to take in. Having to process the fact I had cancer was one thing, but the constant telephone calls from family and friends made the situation even more stressful.

After about ten calls, I was over it. I couldn't tell my story one more time...*at least I didn't want to*. It was exhausting. It kept me in a place where I really didn't want to be. Having to tell my story over and over again made it real and I wasn't mentally ready to accept it yet.

Don't get me wrong, I appreciated the love. I knew people were concerned and wanted to know how I was dealing with my diagnosis, but it was draining to have to constantly repeat myself. I know you are probably thinking, *Why didn't you just stop answering the phone?* The answer is I'm just too nosey. I was hoping that maybe, just maybe, the next call wouldn't be about me having cancer for a change.

One of my dear friends, Justine, suggested I create a blog to keep my family and friends informed of my journey so I wouldn't have to repeatedly share the details. What a great idea! I decided to take heed to her suggestion and I blogged throughout my battle. Prior to my diagnosis, I didn't know much about breast cancer and all that is involved in fighting this battle. However, I knew I had to become a quick learner. After talking to others, I realized I wasn't the only one who didn't know much about breast cancer or what was involved in surviving it. I decided to use the blogs to educate others as I was being taught.

Before I share my blogs with you, let me take you

back in time...just a little. I want to give you a quick glimpse of my life just before this crazy ordeal happened.

Just like the previous years, I brought in 2009 no differently. I started my 2008 New Year Eve's festivities by going to church and then ending the night visiting with family and friends. I was looking forward to the year in which I was turning 39 years old. It was my last year in my thirties before I hit the big 4-0. Life had been great! I was single, had a great career, traveled all over the world. I was loving this adventure called life.

On New Year's Day, I decided to make my resolutions for the upcoming year. I tried to set some achievable goals *in my mind*. The goals were only *in my mind* because I'd learned from past experiences, making resolutions could set me up for major disappointment when I didn't achieve them.

Zig Ziglar, a well-known motivational speaker once said, "A goal casually set and lightly taken is freely abandoned at the first obstacle." Evidently, I hit my first obstacle within the first two weeks of the year because by January 15th, I was no longer focused on those things I resolved. Instead, I decided I was just going to try to make this year my best year yet, even without the resolutions.

In April, I joined Facebook. LOL. LOL = Laughing Out Loud (just in case you didn't know). I know joining social media doesn't seem like a big deal, but it was to me. This platform was a way to connect with people I hadn't seen in years and keep in touch with others. Up to that point, I hadn't had much experience with social media, but a lot of my friends had joined Facebook, so I decided to as well. I wasn't sure of the role social media would play in my life, but it seemed exciting.

During the first week of May, I took a road trip to the Kentucky Derby in Louisville. Going to the Derby was something I always wanted to experience. My friends and I drove down to Louisville on Friday morning, and after the four and one-half hours trip, we arrived at our hotel. We checked in and then went for a quick bite to eat. Afterward, we took a nap so that we would be well rested for the party that night.

We attended a party that was hosted by Tom Joyner, the radio host of the nationally syndicated The Tom Joyner Morning Show. By the time we arrived, Tom Joyner was already leaving the party, however there were other celebrities still partying. For me, one of the best celebrity sightings was Lance Gross, an actor on the TV sitcom *Tyler Perry's House of Payne*. As a former track athlete, I could appreciate his tall, lean build. His skin was reminiscent of chocolate fondue: smooth, rich and creamy. His perfect smile flashed like the sun against the midnight skies. He was just beautiful.

After the late night of partying, we woke up bright and early to attend the race. We all put on our derby hats and headed over to Churchill Downs, the world's most legendary racetrack. We sipped on Mint Juleps, wagered on the races, and enjoyed people watching. I won a whopping $12. It was so much fun. It brought back great childhood memories of when I would go to the horse races in Cleveland with my uncle. However, this was different. This was the Kentucky Derby.

It was during this trip I was given a lesson on the correct pronunciation of the city, Louisville. People from Louisville are offended if you don't pronounce their city correctly. Do you know how to pronounce it? Is it pronounced LOOEYVILLE? *No.* What about LOUIS-VILLE? *Not even close.* LOO-A-VUL? *Yes.* LOO-A-VILLE? *Maybe.* I felt I should use this opportunity to share and have a teachable moment. I hope you enjoyed the lesson.

At the end of June, I had to travel to Dallas for work. My co-workers and I had volunteered to help with the Juvenile Diabetes Research Foundation's summer camp for kids who were battling Type 1 diabetes. Type 1 diabetes, also known as juvenile diabetes is diagnosed in children and young adults. At the camp, we played games, ate great food, and educated the families about my company's insulin pumps and their use in juvenile diabetes. Even though the temperature outside was well over one hundred degrees, it was such an inspiring and uplifting time hanging out with the children. The kids were able to escape their reality, enjoy themselves, and be celebrated.

After the long and exhausting day of being in the sweltering sun with the kids, my co-workers and I headed back to the hotel where we were staying. It was during the ride back that I received the phone call from a friend who said that Michael Jackson had died. "What?!? This can't be true!"

We rushed back to the hotel and to see if the rumor was true. I turned on CNN and MSNBC and they had not reported Michael's death yet. Maybe, just maybe, this was a hoax. At this point, TMZ was the only media outlet reporting that he had died. I remained optimistic for a few hours until it was confirmed that Michael Jackson had died from a drug overdose. My first thought was, *NO! NO!! NO!!! This can't be true.* I'd loved him and his music ever since I was a child. In my mind, we grew up together. Plus,

I had already made plans to see him at his "This Is It" tour in London. I'd purchased my ticket for the opening show on July 8th. My roundtrip airplane ticket had been purchased and my hotel room had been secured.

It was during this time I felt the sporadic pain I had been experiencing for a couple of weeks. I thought to myself, *Ouch! What is this pain I'm feeling? It must be my heart since it's so heavy after learning about Michael's death. Wait a minute, my heart isn't located in my right breast. I need to find out what's going on.*

Although I had planned my trip to London mainly to attend Michael Jackson's concert, I couldn't let his death ruin my vacation. A couple of weeks later, my friend and I continued with our plans to travel to the United Kingdom in July.

It was my first time in London. We visited all the tourist locations: The Parliament, Buckingham Palace, Kensington Palace, Big Ben, museums, the London Eye, London Bridge, and many more attractions. It was a good time seeing all these places I had only seen on television. We also went to see a play, *Dirty Dancing*, which was also playing on Broadway.

Since there wasn't going to be a MJ concert, my friend and I decided to use that extra time to travel to Paris via the Eurostar. The Eurostar is a high speed train that travels under the English Channel to mainland Europe. After we arrived in Paris, we went to the Louvre Museum to see the Mona Lisa, visited the Eiffel Tower, cruised the Siene River, shopped on the Avenue des Champs-E'lysees, took an adventure on their Metro, ate crepes, and was yelled at by a Frenchwoman because we were speaking English.

We even went on an escapade looking for the statue, "The Thinker." This statue, sculptured by Rodin, is a nude man sitting on a rock with his chin resting on one of his hands. He's called The Thinker because...well, he seems be in deep thought. This was an exciting adventure, especially since neither of us had spoken French since high school. By the time we found "The Thinker," the Rodin museum had closed. However, we were able to see the statue through the gates. The security guard was kind enough to take a close-up picture of it for us.

It was good times, nice memories, a great trip.

After recuperating from my trip to London and Paris, I celebrated my 39th birthday with family and friends. I had a beautiful pink and green "basket weave" cake. As I thought about my birthday, I had to ask myself, "Where did the time go?" I mean, for real. It seemed like I had just turned 30 last year. Oh well, I was not going to complain because I'd made it to another year. I still had one more year until the BIG 4-0. Whoo Hoo!

I began thinking about how I could get into tip-top shape by the time I turned 40 years old. I resolved that I would begin a new exercise regimen once the summer was over. I was committed to transform my body to how it was when I was a track star in high school. I didn't want to go back to my high school weight, but I did want my muscles to be defined again.

In September, I started the exercise program, P90X. "I can do it! I can do it! I can do it!" I had to repeat those words to myself for motivation every day as I exercised. After the first couple of weeks, I began to notice changes. I was feeling good about my health; my stamina, strength, and flexibility had improved tremendously. I was proud because I did this without an accountability partner. It was only my desire to be fit that kept me focused and on track.

September was also around the time I was due to have my annual exam. I was searching for a new GYN practitioner. I loved my former gynecologist, but she had stopped practicing medicine. A couple of years prior, she was diagnosed with breast cancer. She was relatively young when this happened; I'm not sure how young, but when I first met her when

I was 19, she was in her late 20's, early 30's. Besides dealing with cancer, she had a husband and a small child to worry about. As you can imagine, it was a very scary time for her. Eventually, she came back to work part-time, but her outlook on life had changed, hence her priorities. She decided she wanted to spend more time doing what she loved the most and that was being with her family. My gynecologist decided to give up her practice and retire.

Even though she's not my gynecologist anymore, I am forever grateful for her because she was the one who encouraged me to start getting mammograms at the age of 30. She suggested the annual mammograms after my sister passed from cancer. Since we never knew where my sister's cancer originated, my doctor felt that it was better to be safe than sorry.

My doctor and I had been together for almost twenty years and I trusted her and valued her opinions. When my doctor sent the letter informing us that she was retiring, she also gave us a list of recommended gynecologists. I didn't know one doctor from another, so I decided to call one of the offices and find out who had the best reputation. After speaking to the receptionist and getting her opinion, I decided to try something new. I made an appointment to see a midwife. At that time, I didn't even know that midwives saw patients who weren't pregnant. My limited knowledge of what they did was that they assisted pregnant women with their childbirths. I knew this seemed like a stretch for a replacement for my doctor, but after asking questions, I thought the midwife might be a really good fit for me.

When I met with the midwife, I mentioned to her I'd been having some pains in my breast for a few months. She performed a breast examination and noticed a lump in my right breast. Seemingly concerned, she gave me a referral so that I could get an ultrasound right away. Still, I wasn't too worried about the lump that she had found because I'd had lumps in my breast for years. My breast tissue was very dense and every year I would be referred to have an ultrasound to make sure the lumps were just breast tissue. Plus, like I told you before, I'd already done a self-diagnosis of the pain I was having in my breast. I had researched it on the worldwide website, AnythingYouWannaKnow.com. Okay, this is a fictitious website, but you get the point. You can pretty much find any information you want on Internet, whether accurate or not.

According to the Internet, the shooting pains in my breast was due to a fibroadenoma, a benign (noncancerous) tumor. They are usually found in women under 30 years of age and African-American women are more likely to develop them. Typically, they are painless, but some can cause pain. I was comfortable with my diagnosis. So, the midwife noticing a lump in my breast was not of concern to me.

Since my new practitioner was affiliated with the Cleveland Clinic, I decided to go to their breast center because they specialized in what else, breasts! A few days later, I had the ultrasound performed. After the reading of the images, a doctor from the breast center called to tell me they saw "something" on the images and that she wanted me to come back and have a biopsy.

No problem, I thought to myself. I'd been through this part before, too. The earliest they could get me in for the biopsy was October 6th, which was a couple of weeks away.

Before the biopsy, I took a solo vacation to Myrtle Beach, SC. I needed to get away for a few days to relax and enjoy the company of myself. I used this time to exhale and reflect on what was next in my life. Where did I see myself going? How was I going to get there? Those were the types of questions I was trying to answer. I would wake up, meditate and watch the sunrise. Afterward, I spent my days on the beach and my nights enjoying dinner and the movies. It was very relaxing having the time to myself and not having to worry about anyone else

or their needs/desires. I had an amazing time enjoying the company of Andrea.

Even while I was on vacation, I remained focused
and disciplined when it came to my workouts. I continued with my P90X routine each day. I was determined to get that six pack...okay, maybe not, but I
did want to tone my stomach.

After returning from South Carolina, it was
finally time to get my breast biopsy. I had shared this
with only a couple of friends because I didn't believe
there was a need for others to be concerned.

The morning of the biopsy, my best friend,
Jackie, asked me if I wanted her to come with me.

I told her, "No, I'll be okay. This is just routine."

I went to breast center to have the lump biopsied.
After it was performed, I was somewhat confused
by the way the doctor and nurses were treating me.
They were rubbing me, hugging me, and telling me
everything would be alright even if the results determined that it was breast cancer.

Two days after the biopsy, my doctor called to
tell me that the results from my biopsy came back
positive.

I was confused, especially since I thought I
already knew the cause of the lump in my breast.
This was not the news I thought I would be hearing.
All of a sudden, I began to think, *How am I going*

to tell my mom? I didn't even know if I could formulate the words. As her only child, I knew this would break her heart. I couldn't imagine the sadness she would feel knowing that I was going through this and that her child could possibly die from this disease.

I thank God for Jackie, because I couldn't have done it without her. Actually, I didn't do it at all. After my diagnosis, I called Jackie and told her the news. She left work and met me at my house so she could take me to my mother's house. Once we arrived, I couldn't bring myself to say anything. I couldn't even look at my mom's face knowing that the words she was about to hear were going to crush her.

I sat on the couch, crying while waiting for Jackie to give her the news. Through her tears, Jackie told her about my biopsy and the results. Surprisingly, my mom handled it much better than I thought she would. Even though she was completely caught off guard, she seemed to take the news okay.

She looked at me and said, "We'll get through this."

My mom's strength made me strong and I stopped crying immediately. At that moment, I felt much better about my situation.

Waiting for my appointments and further testing to take place was difficult. I didn't know how to process everything in my mind. Time could not pass fast enough. I still had the grimacing pain in my breast, and the pain seemed to be more frequent and more intense after the biopsy. I couldn't say for sure — it could have been that I was more aware of the pain because now I knew it was cancer. The mind can be tricky like that. However, I believe that the biopsy disturbed the tumor and that caused the pain to be more frequent and more intense. That sharp, stabbing pain was a constant reminder that I had breast cancer.

It was scary. My mortality was real. There were times when I would sit in my home and look around at all my *things*. These *things* were no longer important to me...not even my baby grand piano. Can I just say it's an upright baby grand with gold trimming and mahogany accents? It's beautiful. I only share this with you because I was so excited when I bought it. Back then, I was starting lessons again. I'd always wanted to be a pianist, or at least be able to play Stevie Wonder's song, "Ribbon In The Sky."

Unfortunately, this new outlook on life caused me to look at my piano differently. It was now just a *thing*. It wouldn't do me any good if I wasn't going to be around long enough to play it. Stuff was just that...stuff. What mattered the most to me wasn't the things I could buy. What mattered were the relationships that I had with my family and friends. That was what was going to help me get through this.

Prior to my diagnosis, I had limited dealings with or knowledge about cancer. Although, there were a few close people in my life who had been affected by cancer, I still didn't know much about the disease. My half-sister, Crystal, was diagnosed with cancer in late 1998 at the age of 40. She was my favorite sister. She and I had a special bond because we were the most similar. I would be so full of pride when people would say how much I reminded them of her. She was tall, beautiful, and super smart.

One day she went into the hospital for surgery and a few months later we were told that she had cancer in all of her organs. Everything seemed to happen so fast. She passed away in April 1999, four months after her diagnosis.

Fortunately, I had a chance to spend time with her before she passed. During our time together, I saw how hard she fought her battle firsthand. I admired her strength and her unwavering faith. She passed away truly believing that she would be healed...*if it was God's will.* She left behind two young children, DJ and Monica. They gave me some peace knowing that I had a piece of her here with me. But still, I missed her dearly.

Then, in December 2000, my grandmother, Katie, was diagnosed with breast cancer after being in a car accident. My grandmother, mom, aunt and I were spending the day doing some Christmas shopping. After shopping, we went to dinner. We had just left Red Lobster and were sitting at a red light when a car hit the front end of passenger's side of our car. The car then sped away. As the driver, I had to chase the hit-and-run driver through the streets and parking lots.

After a while, the driver saw I was still pursuing him and he eventually stopped his car. That was when we found out that he'd been drinking; the driver had just left his friend's bachelor party. The police and ambulance were called. Although none of my family members seemed to be seriously hurt at that time, we decided it would be best to let the ambulance take my grandmother to the hospital, as a precaution.

After each of us gave our statements to the police of how the accident occurred, we drove to the hospital where they'd taken my grandmother. When we arrived, each of us were taken into separate rooms to get checked as well. After the doctor came into my room and observed me, I went into the room with my grandmother.

When I asked her how she was feeling, she said, "Ann, take a look at the little knot on my boob."

I looked at her, then at the knot and said, "Grandma, this isn't a little knot!"

The "little knot" in her breast was the size of my fist...and I have a pretty big fist. I would say it was the size of a small grapefruit or large orange. I told the doctor about this and she suggested we follow up with her family doctor as soon as possible. The next day, we scheduled an appointment with her doctor. After meeting with him, he referred her to a surgeon. The following week she had a mastectomy.

My family was also touched by cancer when my aunt Paula was diagnosed with leukemia. Leukemia is cancer of the blood cells. Most blood cells form in the bone marrow. In leukemia, cancerous blood cells form and crowd out the healthy blood cells in the bone marrow.

I remember the day she was diagnosed like it was yesterday. It was early November, 2007 and I had attended a fund-raising scholarship banquet in downtown Cleveland. As I was leaving the banquet, I received a call from my mom telling me that Paula was being admitted to hospital. My mom told me that earlier in the day, Paula had gone to see her doctor and had a routine blood draw. That evening, her doctor called and told her to go the hospital immediately. Once she had arrived at the hospital, she was told about her condition. She was admitted to the hospital that night and never came home again.

The doctors performed a bone marrow biopsy on her to see which type of leukemia she had so that they could determine how to treat it. She was found to have an aggressive form of leukemia, acute myeloid leukemia (AML).

Every day, our family would visit with Paula. It was like a mini family reunion every time. We would sit around, share stories, laugh, and pray together.

Paula was in great spirits and didn't even look as though she was battling leukemia. However, after two weeks of being in the hospital, her doctor shared the bad news with my uncle. Her doctor told him that my aunt only had six weeks to live.

As you can imagine, we all were shocked and in disbelief. We didn't give much credence to the doctor's prognosis because Paula didn't look sick nor did she act sick. He must not have known what he was talking about. Plus, as Christians, we understood that God was in control and that He could perform a miracle and spare her life...*if it was His will.*

We prayed relentlessly for total and complete healing.

But then, by the fourth week, we could see the cancer slowly taking her away from us. All she asked was for God to give her five more years to spend with her family. As we watched her health quickly decline, we went from asking God to spare her life to asking if He would give her peace and not let her suffer much longer.

Although, the outcome wasn't what the family wanted it to be, it was amazing seeing how God transformed us through her situation. During the process, He had prepared our hearts for what was to come. We went from being in denial and angry about the situation, to being at peace with it. I am grateful that God allowed us to have the time with her during her last days. We were able to let her know what she meant to us and how much we loved her. She passed away six weeks after her diagnosis.

That was the extent of my intimate knowledge cancer, though I did know a few other people who had gone through it, too. I'd known some people who had survived their battles and others who had lost theirs.

As for me, I didn't know what my cancer diagnosis meant for my life, but I knew I had to give it to

God. Trust that He would heal me of this affliction and allow me to use this experience as a testimony of His grace and mercy. I knew with my faith, I already had the victory. Still, I had to get ready to fight with all might.

Here's my journey...

Reflection Questions

1. *What previous plans did you have that became interrupted?*
2. *Who were you before you embarked on your own journey?*
3. *What are your should've/would've/could'ves?*

3

I'm choosing faith

THIS IS THE VICTORY THAT CONQUERS THE WORLD —
OUR FAITH. SO THE ONE WHO WINS AGAINST THE
WORLD IS THE PERSON WHO BELIEVES THAT JESUS IS
THE SON OF GOD.

— 1 JOHN 5:4-5

_____

TUESDAY, OCTOBER 20, 2009 9:03 PM; 12 days
since my diagnosis.

So here I am, almost two weeks since my diag-
nosis, and I'm anxiously waiting to find out more

about my next steps. I'm ready to begin the journey to becoming cancer-free. I still don't know anything about my cancer yet. I haven't been told any information about the type of breast cancer, the size of the tumor, the aggressiveness of the tumor, nor the staging of the tumor.

Tomorrow, I will have my first appointment since the diagnosis. I am scheduled to get an MRI to see if the cancer has spread anywhere else. It's been very difficult not knowing anything. However, I won't get those results until next week when I meet with the surgeon. The results will help determine what my next steps will be. I am just happy that something is finally happening. I'm ready to begin this process so that it can be over with.

I have been very anxious and nervous about the unknown. However, I am thankful I've been able to sleep at night. I've been praying for peace and that is where I am right now, at peace. Well, I was until last night. I didn't sleep well at all. That was the first time I've been restless and I think it's because the MRI is coming up tomorrow. Subconsciously, I think it's affecting me more than I realize.

Besides the breast pain I'm experiencing, the hardest part for me is worrying about how my family and friends are dealing with the situation. I do not like inflicting worry on anyone. I am especially concerned about my mom. She tries to be so strong for me and I appreciate that, but I know she's having a hard time dealing with this, too. Also, it's still tough telling people about the cancer. Saying the words is painful because it makes it real...as if it isn't already.

During this time, my friends and family have been amazing. I know it's also difficult for them, but they have definitely been a great support to me. The prayers and telephone calls are truly appreciated.

Thank you for caring enough to take this journey with me and read my blog. I love each and every one of you. I will leave with you this following psalm. Most of you are familiar with it already, but it's so meaty with God's graciousness, that I had to share.

Psalm 23 (KJV)
[1] The Lord is my shepherd; I shall not want. [2] He maketh me to lie down in green pastures: he leadeth me beside the still waters. [3] He restoreth my soul: he leadeth me in the paths of righteousness for his name's sake. [4] Yea, though I walk through the valley of the shadow of death, I will fear no evil: for thou art with me; thy rod and thy staff they comfort

me. [5] *Thou preparest a table before me in the presence of mine enemies: thou anointest my head with oil; my cup runneth over.* [6] *Surely goodness and mercy shall follow me all the days of my life: and I will dwell in the house of the Lord forever.*

WEDNESDAY, OCTOBER 21, 2009 3:49 PM; 13 *days since my diagnosis.*

Today, I went to get my MRI. Once again, I didn't sleep well last night. I was pretty anxious to have it done. My mom, Aunt Lois, and Jackie, went to the hospital with me. Upon arrival, I checked in and ten seconds later they took me to the back to get the MRI. As I sat there, I just shook my head. I can't believe that I'm going through this. THIS IS ABSOLUTELY CRAZY TO ME!!! It's so surreal. I feel like I'm just going through the motions.

After the technician put an IV in my arm, I was taken into a room and put on the table. As I lie there, I began to pray that cancer wouldn't be found anywhere else in my body. The technician injected contrast into the IV so that it would enhance the images. The scan only took about twenty minutes.

Once the MRI was done, I went back to the waiting room. Jackie said I looked a mess. I probably did.

She thought I had been crying while I was back there, but I hadn't. There was a brief moment when I was about to cry, but it passed and I was able to regroup. We left the hospital and went to the Cheesecake Factory for lunch. Yummy.

I didn't think I would receive any information regarding the results until my meeting with the surgeon next week. However, a few hours after the scan, I received a call on my home phone. Typically, I don't ever bother to answer my home phone, but for some reason I did this time. It was the radiologist calling.

She said she was reading my images and wanted me to come back for another ultrasound before I met with the surgeon. I don't know what all this means. I'm praying that it isn't something else to be concerned about. I can't even waste energy worrying because I know it's impossible to have faith and fear occupying the same space. I'm choosing faith. The good news in all of this is the doctor didn't see anything on the left breast. Praise God for any good news. I am just ready to find out what's next. Right now my nerves are a mess.

A little while later, I received yet another call. This time it was from the surgeon's office. Automatically, I thought it was something bad. However, they were only calling to change the time of my next appointment.

Again, I received another call from the doctor's office, and once again I thought it was something bad. This time, it was about scheduling my ultra-sound. I am going to drive myself crazy with all of these phone calls. I AM A MESS! I have to trust God through this and keep it moving. Otherwise, I may turn into a nut case.

THURSDAY, OCTOBER 22, 2009 9:38 PM; 14 days since my diagnosis.

Even though today has been okay for the most part, I still have my moments. This is serious and very scary. Sometimes I can "forget" I have cancer as I go through my day. But when I sit still, I'm reminded of my situation and I try to process it all. I do believe that I am going to get through this, though. At least that's what I keep telling myself. I think I just need a good cry and then some good sleep.

I was trying to decide if I should even write today, but I felt as though I should say something. I need this blog to help keep my sanity, but I also need to use this platform as a way to make sure people are aware of this breast cancer thing and all that goes along with it after diagnosis. The reality is that this can happen to anyone. Unfortunately, it's me at this time. But, I need to find my purpose while I'm going through this. There is a reason for this. I didn't think I fit the "profile" of someone who would get breast cancer. I am young-er, healthy, fit, and I don't have big boobs. What I've learned is that there really isn't a profile. There are so many people with breast cancer; young and old, healthy and unhealthy, fit and unfit, little boobs and big boobs.

Unfortunately, everyone is at risk for breast cancer. I want to say to all of you out there, please make sure you do your monthly breast exam. I know you hear this all the time, but it is necessary. Women, please don't take your breasts for granted. Men, check your breast tissue, too.

In all the years I walked in the Susan G. Komen's Race for the Cure in honor of my grandmother, never did I think I may have to walk one day in honor of myself. Through God's grace, my grandmother is still here eight years later. I just have to believe I have her strength, too, and that I will still be around eight years from now...with two breasts. But know, if they have to take 'em, adios, boobs.

The tip of the day: Get familiar with your

breasts. *Do your monthly exam religiously. Also, pay attention to your body. Listen to it. Remember, I didn't necessary feel a lump in my breast, but I had pain which is what made me investigate more. Here are four steps to Breast Health Awareness:*

- *Know your risk. Does your family have a history of breast cancer?*
- *Get your breast examinations and mammograms regularly.*
- *Check your boobs monthly. Know how they look, feel and what's normal for you. If you notice a change, follow-up with your doctor.*
- *Make healthier lifestyle choices. Eat more fruit and vegetables.*

SUNDAY, OCTOBER 25, 2009 2:24 PM; *17 days since my diagnosis.*

Here it is, Sunday afternoon. Three days since my last posting. I have given myself permission not to blog every day. Some days, I really don't want to talk about cancer. Yesterday was one of those days and it ended up being a good day. I went to the lunch, went to the movies, and then had visitors. First, my friend Leighton, whom I call Neighbor, came by to visit. He is one my dear friends from college. Even though we weren't necessarily friendly in college, we became friends a few years later when we lived two doors down from each other. Hence the nickname "Neighbor." Even though we haven't been neighbors in over fifteen years, we both still call each other by that nickname. Even his children call me "Auntie Neighbor." LOL.

Anyway, when he arrived at my house, he brought in a package that had been sitting on my front porch. I looked to see who had sent it. It was from one of my co-workers. When I opened the package, there was a gift bag enclosed that read, "It's not what you go through in life – it's how you look while you're going through it!" I had to chuckle because as women, we can be so vain at times.

The other side of the bag read, "A joyful heart makes a cheerful face." – Proverbs 15:13. Reading those words put a smile on my face. Inside the bag, there was a very nice card and a box. I opened the box and saw these beautiful, lavender-colored rosary beads. Since the color of the beads complimented the grey sweater that I was wearing, I decided to take them out of the box and put them around my neck.

I'm not sure what took so long for him to say something, but about forty-five minutes later, Neighbor said, "*Uhh, Andrea, I don't think you're supposed to wear rosary beads around your neck.*"

We both busted out laughing.

"*First of all, why did it take you so long to tell me this? Secondly, how was I supposed to know what to do with the beads? I'm not Catholic and never attended Catholic school.*"

That was hilarious. After he left, I did a little research on the Internet and saw that I'm supposed to carry the rosary beads with me and not necessarily wear as a necklace. However, in the Medieval times, they did wear the beads. I was very appreciative for this thoughtful gift and for the opportunity to laugh at my ignorance. It had been a while since I laughed so hard.

Also, my childhood babysitter, Vanessa, came by to visit me. It was so nice to see her. My other babysitter, who just happens to be her sister, Valerie also visited with me (by phone). These are the two people who cared for me when I was a baby. Here we are almost 40 years later, and they are still caring for me. If either of you are reading this blog, know that I love you both.

Anyway, I am glad I started to blog. It's been very therapeutic for me. Also, I'm really appreciative for all the love and support I've received. It is truly heart-felt.

I know that in order to get through this, I have to continue to stand on God's word. It's the only way for me to have peace of mind. Isaiah 41:10 (KJV) says:

"Fear thou not; for I am with thee: be not dismayed; for I am thy God: I will strengthen thee; yea, I will help thee; yea, I will uphold thee with the right hand of my righteousness."

I trust His word and receive it.

SUNDAY, OCTOBER 25, 2009 7:45 PM; 17 days since my diagnosis; 5 hours and 21 minutes since last blog.

Today, my day started with me going to church. Just like every Sunday since my diagnosis, I cried like a baby during the service. Every word, song, and prayer seemed as though it was just for me. Afterward, I went to go to the store to pick up a card for Neighbor and his wife, Angel. Their baby girl was having surgery and I know that's a scary time for any parent.

I searched to find the perfect card that expressed my thoughts. I found one that said exactly what I wanted to. As I read it, I realized that the card was *encouraging me. I hope that this card will encourage them as well. I just want to share some of the words from the card.*

With God, every day is a day to begin again – to trust and feel His love for us and know that in all of the confusion, there is a gift to be found.

With God, every day is a day to hope for the best – to believe our prayers are being heard, that good news is on its way, that anything can happen between yesterday and tomorrow.

With God, every day is a day to count our blessings, to remember whose children we are, and what we're capable of through a Father who cares so much.

With God, every day is a day to be made new – to forgive and heal, to do what we can, and leave the rest to God.

– Unknown

I hope these words touched you as well. Even though this is my battle, I know that I'm not fighting it alone. I know we are in this together. I want everyone to take a moment and meditate on those words from the card. All that we go through, fight for, and pray for, is to draw us closer to God. He wants us to trust Him and know that He sits on the throne. I'm just happy to know that in all this craziness, there's a blessing to be found. With God...

MONDAY, OCTOBER 26, 2009 9:19 PM; *18 days since my diagnosis.*

It's one more day until I meet with the surgeon. I am very anxious as you can imagine. I just want to know what's next. Unfortunately, my appointment for the ultrasound isn't until noon and my meeting with the surgeon isn't until 1:30 p.m. This waiting is working my nerves. It has been almost three weeks since I found out about the breast cancer. My prayer is that the ultrasound doesn't reveal anything else. Honestly, I'm really praying for a miracle and that the cancer is totally gone. Unfortunately, the pain is still here, so there's a good probability so is the cancer.

I truly feel blessed during all of this. All of you have been so wonderful, more wonderful than I could have imagined. I will never be able to express how much that means to me. Your strength is rubbing off on me. It amazes me how strong I've been in all of this, especially after going through other cancer experiences with my family. I was pretty much done with cancer and would've been just fine if I never had to have another loved one touched by this, myself included. But here I am.

For the past two nights, I haven't really slept that well. On Saturday night, I dreamt about my surgery. I woke up before they started cutting though. Last night, I tossed and turned all night. I am hoping I can sleep tonight. I'm sure my body is tired, so it will have to give in to the sleep...right? I'm going to try to pray my way to sleep.

TUESDAY, OCTOBER 27, 2009 5:59 PM; 19 days since my diagnosis.

Today, I had to get an ultrasound and meet with the surgeon. Anxiously, I woke up at 5:00 a.m. waiting for my noon appointment. My girlfriend, Jackie picked up my mom and me, and then she drove us to the doctor's office. I was a little nervous, but more ready than anything. I was ready to find out when my surgery will be.

When we arrived, the waiting room was packed. After a few minutes, I was called to the back to have my ultrasound. The doctor wanted to compare something new she had seen on my MRI to that of the cancer. As she looked for the cancer, she couldn't find it.

I thought to myself, "Thank you, Jesus. I'm

healed!" Then to my dismay, she said, "Oh, there it is." I was hoping for that miracle I had prayed for. Along with the cancer, the doctor found a new mass. She stated that the new mass didn't look like cancer. She thought it might be a fibroadenoma. How ironic? That is exactly what I had diagnosed before my biopsy.

Anyway, she wanted to be on the safe side, so she suggested that I have a biopsy performed on the mass. Are you kidding me? I have to go through that pain again? As it was, they scheduled me to have the biopsy performed after the appointment with the surgeon.

I'm not sure exactly how many people are on my medical team, but before I met with the surgeon, I had a discussion with another physician who gave me information about the type kind of cancer I have and the several options for treatment that are available to me.

The type of breast cancer that I have is an infiltrating ductal carcinoma, which means the cancer was in the ducts of my breast, but then broke into the surrounding tissue. The cancer is located in the one o'clock position and is 1.3 cm in size, about the size of *a quarter. The doctor mentioned it is not an aggressive cancer and the likelihood of it returning was low.*

That was great to hear. I welcomed any positive news. Also, the cancer tested positive for estrogen receptors which means I can be treated with drugs after the cancer is removed.

As far as my treatment options, I may be able to have a lumpectomy to surgically remove the tumor followed by radiation, or I can do chemotherapy which will shrink the tumor. Another option is to have a mastectomy. I can have my breast removed and then reconstruction performed using the flap procedure, which is where they take fat from your tummy to build up your breasts; or get breast implants. I still don't know which option the surgeon will recommend.

After my conversation with the doctor about the type of cancer I have, the surgeon entered the room. Finally, this is what I'd been waiting for. I want this cancer gone.

I was thinking I was about to hear what my next steps are. NOT! The surgeon told me that she didn't really want to make a recommendation yet because she wanted to see what the biopsy showed on this new mass. That will help her determine the next steps, whether chemotherapy or mastectomy.

As ready as I was to get the process moving, I couldn't help but to think there has to be something a little more attractive than chemotherapy or a mastectomy. I guess one good thing that would come out of a mastectomy would be that I could upgrade to a DD cup...lol.

I will get my results from the biopsy either Thursday or Friday and then meet with the surgeon again on Friday afternoon.

I am relieved that after not patiently waiting, I finally have some answers. It seems as though it took forever to get to this point. I guess I need to learn patience. The following scripture talks about the importance of being patient in order to be made whole. Thank God for His word.

[2] My brethern, count it all joy when ye fall into divers temptations; [3] Knowing this, that the trying of your faith worketh patience. [4] But let patience have her perfect work, that ye may be perfect and entire, wanting nothing. – James 1:2-4 (KJV)

The New International Version (NIV) reads as follows:

[2] *Consider it pure joy, my brothers and sisters,*
whenever you face trials of many kinds, [3] *because*
you know that the testing of your faith produces per-
severance. [4] *Let perseverance finish its work so that*
you may be mature and complete, not lacking any-
thing. – James 1:2-4

Anyway, I'm going to call it an early night. The biopsy was very uncomfortable even though they kept telling me it wouldn't hurt. That's so not true.

Before I finish my blog, I want to leave you with some memorable moments that occurred during this appointment. I wrote the top ten phrases of the day. They are not in any particular order, but these definitely stood out to me.

1. "You have tattoos?" Don't ask.
2. "You can have both of your breasts removed and get a 20-year-old's boobs." My mom and Jackie were trying to make me feel better about my treatment options.
3. "You have genes of healing like your grandmother." Huh? What exactly are healing genes? Of course, those were supposed to be encouraging words from my mom.

4. *"You're healthy." Really? I have cancer. This isn't being healthy.*

5. *"This is good news about your breast cancer..." Isn't this an oxymoron? Is there anything good about having cancer?*

6. *"We can take the fat from your stomach and make you new breasts." I can get a tummy tuck? Yay!*

7. *"Hopefully you won't have to have the surgery too soon." WHAT? Is it ever too soon to have cancer removed?*

8. *"None of the options sounds fun." Why would anybody think any of the options would be fun?*

9. *"They did say it looked benign, right?" Uhh, no, it's cancer.*

10. *"It's good that the cancer is high up instead of on the side." Huh? Regardless, it's still cancer. I guess I get it. The tumor could've been closer to my lymphatic system and could've spread to other areas.*

I had to find humor wherever I could.

[personal reflection]

Of course, this was a difficult time for me. I wasn't sure what was to come. Was I going to live? If so, how would my life be after surviving this disease? I didn't know the answers. I just knew I had to put my faith in God and trust Him during this time.

I am reminded of a quote by the author Steve Maraboli, "Don't give up! It's not over. The universe is balanced. Every set-back bears with it the seeds of a come-back." Being diagnosed with cancer was just a temporary setback. It was to prepare me for my comeback. I wasn't sure what my comeback was, but I was going to give my all during the battle. I would not just survive it, but thrive afterward. I was not going to count myself out just yet.

Israel Haughton, a gospel musician, has a song called "It's Not Over." The lyrics of the song is a reminder that it's not over when God's in it. The "*it*" can be whatever situation you face. Mine just happened to be cancer. As we know, God has the final say in every situation. We all will face adversities at some point in our lives and we will have to confront them head on. During that time, we must learn to embrace the storms and trust that they are for our good in the end. They will come to teach us and make us more resilient.

In the Bible, there were several instances where

"it" wasn't over. King Nebuchadnezzar of Babylon besieged Jerusalem and took many Israelites captive. Among these were the Hebrew boys, Shadrach, Meshach and Abednego. The king had built a huge golden image and commanded all the people to fall down and worship it whenever they heard the sound of his musical herald. Anyone who did not take heed to his order would be thrown into a fiery furnace.

The three Hebrew boys refused to bow to the golden image and only worshipped the true God. Because of this, they were reported to the king. The king was furious when he heard this and ordered that they be brought to him. He asked them if it was true that they wouldn't serve his god. He ordered them to fall down and worship the golden image again, else be thrown into the furnace immediately.

He asked, "What god will be able to rescue you from my hand."

The Hebrew boys responded, "King Nebuchadnezzar, we do not need to defend ourselves before you in this matter. If we are thrown into the blazing furnace, the God we serve is able to deliver us from it and he will deliver us from Your Majesty's hand."

King Nebuchadnezzar became furious and ordered the furnace to be heated seven times hotter than usual. He commanded his strongest soldiers to tie them up and throw them into the furnace. The furnace was so hot that it consumed the soldiers and the three Hebrew boys fell into the furnace.

The king stood up and asked, "Weren't there three men that we tied up and threw into the fire? Look! I see four men walking around in the fire, unbound and unharmed, and the fourth looks like a son of the gods." (Dan. 3:24-25)

The king called Shadrach, Meshach and Abednego to come out of the fire and they emerged unharmed, with not even a hair on their heads singed or the smell of smoke in their clothing. Although they were put in a fiery furnace, they were not consumed. *It wasn't over...*

Lazarus had been dead in the tomb for four days. His sister Martha said to Jesus, "If you had been here, my brother would not have died. But I know that even now God will give you whatever you ask."

Jesus told her that your brother would rise again. Martha answered that she knew he would rise again in the resurrection at the last day.

Jesus said to her, "I am the resurrection and the life. The one who believes in me will live, even though they die; and whoever lives by believing in me will never die. Do you believe this?" (John 11:25)

Martha called her sister Mary and told her Jesus was looking for her. After seeing Mary weeping over the death of Lazarus, Jesus was deeply moved in spirit and troubled. He asked where they had laid Lazarus. Jesus asked for them to remove the stone where he was buried and called for Lazarus to raise from dead. (John 11:43) *It wasn't over...*

Jesus was crucified, buried, and rose again with all power in His hands. (Matt. 27 and 28) *It wasn't over...*

Sometimes we are so quick to place a period where God has only placed a comma. We may think it is the end, but God is only intending for it to be a pause. We should never discount who God is in our lives and what He can do.

Unfortunately/fortunately, we don't know His plan for us, but His plan is always better than the one we create. We have to keep trusting His word and realize that He has the final say. In reading His word, we have many promises that we can stand on. He promises us that, "I will never leave you nor forsake you." I believe in His word and I will continue to trust Him.

It's not over until God says it's over...

———

Reflection Questions

1. *Think of a time when you experienced a set-back. What were the circumstances?*

2. *What was the come-back that resulted from the set-back?*

3. *How did you use your faith to get through it?*

4

my genes or not my genes?

"YOU DON'T CHOOSE YOUR FAMILY. THEY ARE GOD'S GIFT TO YOU, AS YOU ARE TO THEM."

– DESMOND TUTU

WEDNESDAY, OCT. 28, 2009 7:36 PM; 20 days since my diagnosis.

Today, I went to see the movie "Michael Jackson's This Is It." It was great! However, watching the movie opened some old wounds. I am still very disappointed knowing I was only three weeks away from seeing the concert of a lifetime. I know I can't live in the would've/could've/should'ves, but had he lived just twenty-one more days...

Let me share some good news with you all. Around 5:20 this evening, I received a telephone call from the Cleveland Clinic. Anytime I see the 444, 445, and 839 exchanges in the phone number, my heart drops to the floor. This call was from the doctor who saw the "other" mass on the MRI and performed the biopsy. She said that the other tumor was not cancer. Thank you, Jesus! So now, I only have one cancer mass to focus on. By Friday, I should know my treatment plan and when it starts.

Earlier this morning, the surgeon's office called because the doctor wants me to do genetic counseling. Genetic counseling is the process by which the patients who may be at risk of a genetic condition are advised of the chances of being affected by or having a child or other family member with a genetic condition. My doctor wanted to see if I was a carrier of the BRAC1 or BRAC2 gene. These are the two genes that have been associated with the increased risk of breast and ovarian cancers. Carriers of these genes *account for less than 1 percent of the general popula-tion. If the test comes back that I have either of the two genes, it will change my treatment plan. I would possibly have to have my ovaries removed, too. I can't worry myself about that yet, especially since the test-ing hasn't even be done.*

This has been a roller coaster ride. More downs than ups, but I still have to praise God for any pos-itive news. The waiting and uncertainty is really wearing on me. I have to throw up my hands and give it to God because I know there's a reason I'm going through all of this. Nonetheless, I am feeling better today. I hope I get a good night's rest. I'll blog again on Friday.

[personal reflection]

Even though I didn't think I was a carrier of the breast cancer gene, I was curious to find out what the results were from the genetic testing. At that point, my maternal grandmother was the only other fam-ily member diagnosed with breast cancer. On my dad's side of the family, I'm not aware of anyone else who had breast cancer. As I mentioned earlier, my sister died from cancer that had spread throughout her organs. Unfortunately, we never knew where her cancer originated, so I can't rule out that it may have started with breast cancer.

Up to this point, I haven't mentioned my dad. Yes, he is still a big part of my life. His genes are definitely important when it comes to this testing because he's half of my DNA. My dad now lives in Roanoke, VA, but he lived in Cleveland for the majority of my life. It wasn't until I was 29 years old that my dad left Cleveland to return to his hometown. At this point in my blog, he didn't know about my cancer.

I didn't even know how to tell him, especially because I knew how hard he took it when my oldest sister was diagnosed with cancer. When she became ill, he decided to move back to Virginia to be closer to her. It was only a few months after he moved down there that my sister died. It was a very sad time for my family, but especially for my dad. He loved him some Crystal. She was his first baby girl. Knowing how he handled my sister's death, I couldn't even begin to imagine how my dad would feel once he found out about me having cancer. I was his "baby." I was his youngest child...*as far as I know.* LOL. If you know my dad, then you understand that comment.

Wait, let me share this funny-ish story with you right quick. Don't get me wrong, there is no judgment here. I love my dad. Even though I am my mom's only child, I grew up knowing that my dad had three sons and three other daughters who lived in Roanoke. They were all older than me. I would see them when they came to Cleveland to visit our dad or when I went to Roanoke to visit. Throughout the years, I was able to develop my own relationships with them. However, in the summer of 1994, I met a "new" brother. He is older than me and looks just like my dad. So now, I know of three sisters and four brothers. That makes eight of us, right? However, in 2005, my dad went to his 55th class reunion. He was so excited to tell me that he won the award for having the most kids. I laughed. I mean, eight is a lot of kids. Most people don't have more than two and one-half. Something made me ask him how many kids did he have to have to win such an award.

He told me, "*They* said I have twelve."

I asked, "Twelve? What? Daddy, who are *they*? How would *they* know unless you told them?"

All I could do was shake my head and laugh. My dad is a mess. So, earlier when I made the comment, "as *far as I know*," this is the reason why I said it. I only know of the eight of us but there may be four other siblings out there somewhere. I wish I knew how to find them. Since I grew up as an only child, I love meeting new siblings.

You gotta love my daddy, though. Well, you don't have to, but I do. He has always been so proud of me and did his best to spoil me. When I was in college, he would cook dinner for me every night so I didn't have to eat cafeteria food. He was also responsible for getting me my first summer internship. He met a man who worked at BP Headquarters when it was in Downtown Cleveland. He bragged on me so much that the man asked my dad to forward his information to me. I called and we arranged to meet. When we met for lunch, he told me about a position within the company. The next thing I knew, I was working as a summer intern making good money. I tell you, my dad never met a stranger. He had such a great personality.

As you can see, my dad loved him some Andrea. That's one reason why I couldn't bear having to share my breast cancer diagnosis with him over the telephone. He was going to be devastated. I needed someone to be with him once he found out. My mom called my aunt who also lives in Roanoke and told her about my situation. She went over to my dad's place and told him the news. After he found out, he called me. He seemed to take the news pretty good...well as good as can be expected.

Both my dad and my mom tried to be strong for

me during this time. It's awesome to know how much they love me.

———

Reflection Questions

1. *Are you aware of your family history?*
2. *What are some of your genetic traits that you need to pay attention to?*

5

hurry up and wait

"PATIENCE IS NOT SIMPLY THE ABILITY TO WAIT — IT'S
HOW WE BEHAVE WHILE WE'RE WAITING."

— JOYCE MEYER

———

THURSDAY, OCTOBER 29, 2009 9:04 PM; 21
days since my diagnosis.

*AAAAHHHHHHHHH!!! That's my scream of
frustration. I was hoping the next time I blogged, it
would be after my meeting with the surgeon. Unfortunately, my appointment has been moved from*

tomorrow to next Tuesday. The waiting is slowly driving me crazy. I just wanna cry.

In the meantime, I did some research on the type of cancer I have. There are so many different ways to treat it. I guess I will need to figure out what is the best option for me after my meeting with the surgeon.

TUESDAY, NOVEMBER 3, 2009 5:20 PM; 26 days since my diagnosis.

Today was the day I met with the surgeon...again. While in route to meet me at the office, Jackie called to see how I was doing. I was doing pretty good at this point. However, as I got closer to the doctor's office, I started getting anxious again. My nerves felt like they did when I ran the 400 meters in the Ohio State Championship track meet.

I met my mom at the front door and we walked to the breast center to meet up with Jackie. When we arrived, Leighton (a.k.a. Neighbor) was sitting there with Jackie. What a nice surprise. He didn't even tell me he was going to come to my appointment. I was really excited to have all of them there with me.

We met with the surgeon to find out what I needed to do to get rid of this cancer. I really don't want to do chemotherapy. I had even considered a mastectomy as a way to avoid chemotherapy. Unfortunately, the surgeon gave me a couple of options and both of them included chemo. I could have a lumpectomy or a mastectomy. However, both options still required me to do chemo. I am not looking forward to it, however I am looking forward to being cancer-free. Therefore, I will have to do what I have to do.

I am going to get a second opinion, just to be thorough and help me be more comfortable with the options that were presented. My surgeon gave me the name of a couple of surgeons at University Hospitals of Cleveland.

Meanwhile, I have appointments coming up with an oncologist, a plastic surgeon (just in case I want my DDs), and the genetic counselor. Also, I have an appointment for another procedure. The surgeon wants to put a metal clip on the cancer so they can monitor the reduction of the mass with chemo. The clip will allow them to mark the cancer so even if it shrinks so small that it's difficult to find, they will still know where it was located. Also, I have to make the appointment for the second opinion. These next few weeks are going to be busy, but at least something is happening.

TUESDAY, NOVEMBER 3, 2009 10:47 PM; 26
days since my diagnosis.

*Dear family and friends, I just want to say that I
love you all. I am truly blessed to have so many people in my corner, going through this with me. Thank
you. During this time, I've received various thoughtful gifts from you: an awareness pin, earrings, Pan-
dora charms, breast cancer awareness popcorn,
rosary beads, a bracelet, praying angels, and a glass.
I've also received cards, phone calls, visits, words of
encouragement, scriptures and prayers. You've even
given me shoulders to cry on. For that, I am truly
grateful. You cannot understand how much this
means to me during this time. All of this has made
it easier for me to deal with and accept my situation.
This road hasn't been easy and it will get worse
before it gets better, but your thoughtfulness and
prayers have helped me along.*

*P.S. Knowing that the surgeon wants me to go
through chemo is really bothering me. I don't want
to go through it because I don't know what it means
for me and my body. We've seen the images of people
going through chemo. It is not pretty. Thankfully,
someone just sent this scripture over to me and it definitely made me feel better.*

"Peace I leave with you, my peace I give unto you: not as the world giveth, give I unto you. Let not your heart be troubled, neither let it be afraid." –
John 14:27 (KJV)

I will not be afraid as I go through this process. I will do what I have to in order to survive. I am determined.

––––––––––––

[a quick reflection]

During this time, I was still working. I had to travel to Phoenix for a work meeting. I was hoping to find some time to relax while I was there. While traveling on the plane, there was a lady sitting across the aisle from me who was talking to someone about her weight and nutrition. She mentioned she had gained weight while taking the drug, Tamoxifen. I had to take a look at her. I needed to see what she looked like. Had it been a couple of months prior, I wouldn't have known what Tamoxifen was. Now, I recognized that it is a chemo drug...the same drug I will have to take for five years.

As we deplaned, I asked the lady about her experience with the drug. She said it was her fourth year and the only side effect she experienced was weight gain. I was happy to hear she only had one side effect, but I was aware we all reacted to drugs differently. While I was taking the drug, I hoped the weight didn't decide to stick with me.

Once I arrived in Phoenix, I headed to the hotel with some time to spare. I decided to have a deep tissue massage before the meeting. Lovely. This was exactly what I needed. I was very relaxed afterward. However, during my first night in Phoenix, I had a nightmare. It woke me out of my sleep. I dreamt that I had surgery and they found cancer in my lungs. Lord, help me! Rarely do I experience nightmares. I decided to have a glass of wine to help me fall back asleep.

MONDAY, NOVEMBER 9, 2009 11:45 PM; *32 days since my diagnosis.*

Wow. I can't believe it's been almost a week since I last blogged. I guess I wanted to take some time away. Plus, there hasn't been any new news until today...well, kind of. First of all, I want to thank my cousin/niece/daughter, Teryn, for my cupcakes. She is really my cousin, but I treat her like my niece and I wish she was my daughter. She has such a huge heart and knows exactly how to make me feel better...and get me fat. I desperately need to start my P9oX workout program again.

Having been away from my computer for the past few days, I spent most of this morning catching up on emails. That's when I ran across an email from one of my co-workers. The subject line read "The Grotto at Notre Dame." I wasn't sure exactly what that meant, but when I read the email, I realized that my co-worker had lit a candle in honor of me last Saturday night at the Grotto at Notre Dame University. The lit candle represented a prayer intention. It is so wonderful to know that I have people praying for me even when I can't pray for myself. Of course, as soon as I saw the picture of my candle, I cried. That was so sweet and thoughtful of him.

This afternoon, I finally had my first meeting with the oncologist. I had been waiting for this appointment for a while. I didn't go into the meeting thinking I would be starting chemotherapy treatment today, however I was hoping that I would find out exactly when I would be starting. There are some things I need to get in order before I start chemo. Plus, I am ready to begin because the sooner I begin, the sooner it will be over.

When I met with the oncologist, he performed a

physical exam. He mentioned the mass wasn't that big and he doesn't agree with me doing chemo before removal of the cancer. You may remember that my surgeon preferred for me to do chemo first to shrink the mass and to also treat my whole body. The oncologist's thoughts are that if I do the chemo first, it will get rid of the mass (or most of it) and he would not be able to do any testing on it. He wouldn't be able to stage it, nor would we ever know if the cancer was in my lymph nodes because the chemo would most likely kill all the cancer cells if there were any. Also, if I do chemo first, he would have to give me the most aggressive treatment, even if I don't need it.

After some discussion, my oncologist came up with a solution I was a little more comfortable with, but he needed to discuss it with my surgeon. He suggested I have my lymph nodes removed first so that he would be able to determine what type of treatment I need. He doesn't want me to take more chemo than necessary. Nonetheless, I won't know my next steps until I meet with him again next week. Can you believe that? Still, no answers as to when I will begin treatment yet...

I almost forgot to tell you, while at the appointment, I watched a DVD that described what I should expect from chemotherapy. It was very informative and it made me feel a little more comfortable with having to do this. Also, the nurse went over all the side effects and what I could expect from the respective drugs. I received tons of information and resources and found out about a workshop that teaches how to use a scarf to cover a bald head. I guess I have to come to the realization that I will lose my hair, but at least I'll have my life.

The nurse also showed me the treatment area where I will receive my chemo treatment. They have nice, comfortable reclining chairs, TVs, VCRs, videos, books, and snacks. This will help make the time go by faster as I'm getting the drugs put in my body.

I will keep you informed as to my next steps. Right now it seems like I have appointment after appointment after appointment. I do realize this is just the nature of fighting this disease, but goodness, I'm trying to do everything to not get discouraged or impatient.

FRIDAY, NOVEMBER 13, 2009 10:16 PM; 36 days since my diagnosis.

Since my last entry, I've had two more doctor

appointments, one with the plastic surgeon and one to have the clip put into the tumor. The plastic surgeon's appointment was a little premature. I'm not even sure I will be needing him. However, the doctor gave me some information about the various procedures that are available. He talked about the reconstruction surgery where they take fat from the stomach area to make a new breast.

He looked at my stomach and said, "I see you have enough fat to get enough tissue for a new breast."

Did he just say that? Did he really just say that? I guess I need to do some ab work...quickly. He told me to come back once I was sure that I will have reconstruction surgery. I took the various brochures and left.

Next, I was off to the appointment for the placement of the clip. I was nervous about this one because every time the tumor is disturbed, I end up in a lot of pain.

When I entered the breast center, I realized I was more than just another familiar face. I've been there so many times in the past few weeks that they now know my name. That made me sad. I realized I'm tired of being there and the sad part is I haven't really started battling the cancer yet.

The procedure for inserting the clip was pretty much the same as it was with the biopsy. The nurse who had given me a hug during my first biopsy was there again. She directed me into the room and prepped the area on my breast where the clip would be inserted. Once the doctor came in, she numbed the area so that it wouldn't hurt when they nicked my skin. However, it didn't help when they inserted the clip into the tumor. The pain brought tears to my eyes again. I couldn't stop them from falling no matter how hard I tried. I told the doctor I've had pain all along. She was the only doctor I've talked to who acknowledged that breast cancer can cause pain. Every other doctor seemed to think the pain wasn't from the cancer, but from something else...like it was in my mind. I guess I'm sharing this because I want you all to know that breast cancer can hurt and once again, pay attention to your body.

Well, having three appointments this past week was definitely enough to mentally drain me. I'm glad it's the weekend. I will have a couple of days to rest and relax. Hopefully, I'll get some more answers on

Monday when I meet with the oncologist again. Until the next time...

MONDAY, NOVEMBER 16, 2009 10:14 PM; 39 days since my diagnosis.

Am I entitled to have a bad day? If so, then today is it. I have been on an emotional rollercoaster. I would be okay one minute and then crying the next. It was just one of those days. After work, I went to my appointment with the oncologist. He asked me if I had spoken to my surgeon. I hadn't yet. He said he spoke to her last week and they had agreed with his plan. He thought I should have the lymph nodes removed first so that they can see if the cancer has spread anywhere else. If there's not any cancer cells in my lymph nodes, then I will only have to do four rounds of chemo every three weeks. If they do find cancer cells in the lymph nodes, I will have to do a more aggressive regimen which would be eight treatments every two weeks.

The oncologist said my surgeon's nurse will call me today or tomorrow with an appointment for surgery. He seems to think surgery will happen within the next two weeks. After the surgery, I will have to meet with him again to get the results and then plan *for the chemotherapy. To add to everything else that's going on in my life, my blood pressure was high. I know that's understandable considering everything I'm going through, but I was a little disappointed. My blood pressure had never been high before and I thought I'd been handling this pretty well, not internalizing it so much. I guess not...*

This evening, I went to choir rehearsal. I had all intentions of sharing what I was going through with my choir members. Unfortunately, I couldn't keep myself together. Every song we rehearsed seemed like it was just for me. I couldn't stop crying. I would get up and go to the back of the church to wipe away the tears and then come back and continue to sing. One time, I was crying so hard that I had to go to the restroom to get myself together. Some of the children of the choir members were in there.

One of my favorite church-children looked at me with concern and asked, "What's wrong? Are you okay?"

At that moment, all I could do is wipe my tears, give her a hug, and tell her I was okay. I ran out of there as fast as I could. I didn't want to concern the kids with my issues.

My choir director knew what I was going through

because of our mutual friend. When rehearsal was almost over, she asked me if I wanted to say anything to the choir members. I told her no because I didn't feel like crying in front of everyone. She asked if it was okay if they prayed for me.

After the prayer, my director asked if everyone could come to the altar and close rehearsal with the song "Be Blessed" by Bishop Paul Morton. If you know me, then you know I boo-hooed all the way up to the altar. I think I need to pause right here and just say to all my cousins out there, do not use this as an opportunity to make a joke about me being a cry baby with a runny nose as a kid. Please and Thank you.

Okay, I digressed. Anyway, some of the words to "Be Blessed" are as follows:

You might be hurtin', you might be cryin',
You might be worryin' and frustrated, too.
Let me encourage you.
Let me speak life to you.
You can depend on God to see you through.
You can depend on me to pray for you. [1]

Those words really resonated with me. I am/was hurting. I am/was crying. I am definitely worrying and very much frustrated. I really needed to hear that song. I needed those words. I needed encouragement. This song is definitely going to be in my head and my heart tonight.

God is going to see me through this. I trust Him. I believe He will bring me through this victoriously.

Yes, I am entitled to a bad day. However, even during my bad days, I still have to be thankful. Thankful that I woke up this morning. Thankful for all the love and support that has been shown to me. Thankful even for this experience. There is a reason for this. I know I will be a better person once I get through this and I will have a stronger relationship with God because of it.

Okay, it's time for me to get ready for bed. I need a moment to exhale and get my attitude right. Actually, I am feeling much better just by sharing my day with you. Talk to you soon. I still need to blog about my first experience at The Gathering Place, which is a facility that offers programs and services for all those who are touched by cancer. The information about that experience will be coming in a later blog. Love you all.

[personal reflection]

Although some things were happening, it seemed as though the process was moving slowly. Yes, I've had many appointments, but I wanted this cancer out of me. I was still waiting to find out when I was going to have the surgery to see if the cancer had spread to my lymph nodes. Surprisingly, I was ready to start chemo. I needed to feel as though I was actively fighting cancer.

At times, I just wanted to escape from my reality. I was so over this. However, I had to keep pressin' and praisin'. I had to remember not to diminish God because of my situation, but to diminish my situation because of my God.

"Now to him who is able to do immeasurably more than all we ask or imagine, according to His power that is at work within us, to Him be glory in the church and in Christ Jesus throughout all generations, for ever and ever! Amen."- Ephesians 3:20 (NIV)

I will not doubt nor will I put limits on what God can do in my life. I will not insult Him by my small thinking.

Reflection Questions

1. *Can you think of a time when you felt like things were going slower than you would've like?*

2. *How did you handle this situation?*
3. *How did you learn patience in the process?*

6

moving in forward motion

"EVEN IF YOU FALL ON YOUR FACE, YOU'RE STILL MOVING FORWARD."

– VICTOR KIAM

———

TUESDAY, NOVEMBER 17, 2009 9:02 PM; 40 days since my diagnosis.

Finally, I have a date for surgery! It will take place on Monday, November 30th. I will have surgery to remove my lymph nodes to see if any of the cancer cells traveled to the lymph nodes and possibly other sites. As you may recall, this will help determine how much chemotherapy I will receive. Of course, I'm praying for the lesser of the two treatments. The aggressive chemo can affect my organs more than the other. Also, if I have to do the aggressive chemo, I would have to have additional testing done in order to see if my heart would be able to handle it.

THURSDAY, NOVEMBER 19, 2009 8:41 PM; 42 days since my diagnosis.

Today started out pretty good. I woke up early and decided to try to catch up on my work. I needed to tie up some loose ends, especially since my treatment is coming up soon. I turned on my bath water and then took out my garbage.

As I walked back into my garage and passed my truck, I thought to myself, I should scan my inventory for work. My company sells medical devices and typically, we are there in surgery to ensure that the devices work correctly. I keep my products in my trunk so that they are accessible as needed. Periodically, I have to scan my products to do a check and balance on my inventory. This allows me to verify that I didn't misplace/lose any product.

After I scanned my product, I called one of my co-workers to see when we could meet up so I could give her the scanner. Once we set up a time to meet, I headed back upstairs to get dressed.

"What is that noise?" I couldn't figure out what the sound was I was hearing. "Did I leave the radio on? Again, what is that noise?"

As I got closer to my bedroom, I was able to figure it out. It was my bath water. Two and one-half hours after I started running my bath. How could I forget I was running bath water? Fortunately, for me and my home, there's an invisible drain somewhere that didn't let my tub overflow. That would've been a disaster. Two point five hours of water running at full blast. My water bill is going to be ridiculous. Needless to say, I had to wait another hour before my water heated up again so I could take a bath. My bathroom smelled like a swimming pool with all the chlorine that was in the water. I guess this is what stress can do to you. I was totally distracted...

After that near disaster, I received a phone call from the surgery department. They have moved my surgery up from November 30th to November 25th (the *day before Thanksgiving). That's good news, I guess. At least the process is beginning sooner rather than later. Unfortunately, it's the day before my favorite holiday. Hopefully, I'll do fine with the surgery and I'll be able to eat like I want to.*

This process has been something else. There are some things I don't even share in my blog because it just seems like it's too much at times. However, I will share with you that I did go to my genetic counseling appointment yesterday. I am going to have the BRAC analysis done (for those who may have seen the commercial). Basically, this test (analysis) will show if I'm a carrier of the breast cancer gene. The result will definitely affect my decision as I get closer to surgery.

Well, that's it for now...no, wait. The other day, I mentioned I would share my experience at The Gathering Place. This is a facility where those who are touched by cancer can come together and support one another. They provide service to those diagnosed with cancer and their family and friends.

I attended the orientation and was one of three new people who were being oriented to the facility. All three of us had been recently diagnosed with cancer: one person was diagnosed with and breast can-

cer which presented itself in her eyes, one with ovarian cancer, and then myself. Leading the orientation, were two breast cancer survivors. We all had a nice time just being able to talk and share our experiences so far. I was the youngest of the group.

Ironically, both of the other women who were being oriented were Russians. I shared with them that I had visited Russia when I was selected as one of three runners who represented the United States in a Peace Run held in Volgograd, Russia. Just in case you didn't notice, I said Peace Run and not Peace Race because I wasn't racing anyone. My goal wasn't to finish before anyone. It was to just finish. It was a 10K (6.2 miles) that took place with temperatures of 30-40 degrees below zero. Yes, you read it right. Below zero. I had icicles hanging from my eyebrows. Never again.

However, traveling to Russia was a great experience. I had the opportunity to hang out with runners from various communist countries and learn about their cultures. Also, I visited Lenin's tomb located in the infamous Red Square. I waited in line for over three hours, in the cold, to see Lenin's embalmed body for about 10 seconds. Exciting, huh? Not really. This was an experience. I'm not even sure how else to describe it. In case you don't know who Lenin was, he was a Russian communist who was responsible for forming the Soviet Union. Anything more you'd like to know about him, you can find on Google. Okay, I digressed. Let's get back to my time at The Gathering Place.

After sharing my experiences about Russia, the Russian ladies suggested I go back to visit again. They said it has changed a lot. Uhh, not. Even though Moscow was memorable and looked as amazing in person as it does on TV, I don't have a desire to go back. I politely let them know there were too many other places in the world that I haven't visited yet.

Despite the circumstances that brought us together at The Gathering Place, it was great to create a bridge of cultures that otherwise would have not been built. That is one of the things that makes The Gathering Place awesome. In addition to that, the facility offers support groups, exercise classes, art classes, and massages. The best part of it all is that it's free.

I didn't know what to expect, but I'm glad I went. I enjoyed meeting other people going through the same thing. I thought I was going there to see how the center could help me, but I found myself helping and encouraging others along in their journey. I realized that there were some people who go through this battle without hope. There were people who didn't have any faith to lean on during this difficult time. I don't know how they do it because it seems so dark and depressing. Personally, I choose to follow the Light. I choose to put my faith in the Lord and let Him lead me along the way.

I was able to share tips that I found to be helpful. For instance, I suggested they take a recorder with them to their doctor's appointments, especially for the lady who didn't speak English well. Sometimes when I went to my appointments, it was hard to process everything the doctor said. I would hear something and began focusing on that one thing. I would end up missing other pertinent information. I noticed when I reviewed my appointments via the recorder, there were some things that I totally missed or forgot was said. It helps to be able to go back and listen to the appointments again.

There was also a library at The Gathering Place. It has every book you could imagine regarding cancer. The library staff recommended that I read Dr. Susan Love's, Breast Book. I didn't need a library card or any identification. All I had to do was take the index card out of the back of the book, put my name with the date on it. I was told I could return the book at my leisure. How cool is that? I was glad to hear I could return it whenever, because it's a pretty thick book.

On the monthly schedule of activities, I saw a workshop that I wanted to attend, "Look Good...Feel Better." This program is supported by the American Cancer Society. I can't wait to attend because I desperately need to look good and feel better. I will let you know how it goes.

SUNDAY, NOVEMBER 22, 2009 4:43 PM; 45 days since my diagnosis.

Since my last update, I've had my second opinion. Basically nothing that was said is going to change my next steps. Still chemo, and then the removal of the tumor. When I met with the surgeon at University Hospitals of Cleveland, he pretty much said the same thing my oncologist said. He thought the cancer should be taken out first just to get more information. I understood his thoughts, but that would lead to my breast possibly being deformed; my original surgeon is trying to preserve my breast. This surgeon made a point that it wouldn't matter if it were deformed if I were planning to have a mastectomy, but that decision hasn't been made yet. I still need to get the results from my genetic counseling to help determine how I will move forward.

I'm trying to take it one step at a time. I don't want to stress myself out too much. The surgeon agrees with having the lymph nodes removed first to see what I can find out. He even suggested I get them biopsied before the surgery. This could possibly eliminate the need for surgery if cancer is found. I decided to do the biopsy to see if I could save myself from a surgery. The process involved having an ultrasound of my lymph nodes under my arm and seeing if anything looks unusual. If so, they would test that particular lymph node and see what information they could get from it.

During the ultrasound, they saw one lymph node that looked a little different than the others so they decided to biopsy it. If it has cancer cells, I would have to start with the more aggressive chemo since that would mean that the cancer had spread.

Prayerfully, the lymph node will not contain any cancer cells. I won't get the results until Monday or Tuesday. I made sure the doctors were aware my surgery was scheduled for Wednesday and I needed the results expedited.

This biopsy was more painful than I anticipated. Unlike the needle used for the breast biopsy, which was the size of a pencil, this needle was much smaller yet more painful.

I thought to myself, "Why did I do this biopsy? Most likely I'm going to have surgery anyway."

I don't believe I'm thinking logically at times. It made sense to me at some point, but now it doesn't. It was difficult for me to drive or do anything with my right arm afterward.

On Saturday, I had to get the H1N1 flu (a.k.a. swine flu) vaccination. My doctor recommended it since my immune system was going to be suppressed. At this time, they were only allowing people who are considered high risk to be given the vaccine, and unfortunately, I fell into that category. When I arrived at the center to get my vaccination at 9 a.m., there was an extremely long line. Everybody was scared of this H1N1, especially those parents with small children. It took about thirty minutes for me to make it through the line and get my shot. Now, I'm prepared with both the regular flu and the H1N1 vaccinations. As you know, this will be important for me when I start chemo since I won't have much of an immune system to fight off anything.

I was happy things were starting to taking place. This made me a little anxious, though. However, I'd been receiving many cards which had helped me stay encouraged. I was tickled when I opened my mail and received the same card I had bought for Neighbor and his wife, Angel when their daughter was having surgery. Now, I had it in hard print for myself. Anyway, I just have to share again. I won't write out the entire card, but I will share the following stanza:

With God, every day is a day to begin again – to trust and feel His love for us, and know that in all of the confusion, there is a gift to be found...

There is a gift to be found in all of this. I just can't wait to figure out what it is. I can't wait until it reveals itself to me.

Also on Saturday, my cousin Terri, who's a professional photographer, took some pictures of me. I wanted to have pictures to remember what I looked like before I started my battle. I know the person I was before cancer will never be again and I wanted to have a picture to remember the old me.

TUESDAY, NOVEMBER 24, 2009 10:08 PM; 47 days since my diagnosis.

Tomorrow is the day! I am eating and drinking all the way up until midnight. I have to be at the surgery center at 7:30 a.m. and my surgery is scheduled for 8:30. As you may recall, I did the node biopsy last week to see if I had cancer in the nodes. The results came back negative. That's a good thing, but I still have to go through with the surgery just to ensure there is not cancer in any of the other nodes. They told me the surgery should only last about an hour and one-half. I pray I recover fast and I'm out of there by noon.

They shared with me the road to recovery after surgery wasn't going to be easy. After the removal of the nodes, there's a chance that my shoulder can become stiff. Therefore, I will have to start physical therapy to ensure it doesn't become a problem for me. Also, I may need a drain to rid the wound of excess fluid. I'm hoping I don't, but if I do, that will affect some things. I wouldn't be able to drive until it's out (in about two weeks), plus I will have to empty it out periodically and log the amount of fluid that drains from it. I realize this is surgery, but I guess I didn't know all that would be involved. I found out that *once the lymph nodes are gone, I can never give blood from that arm again. Whew.*

Before I sign off, I just want to say Happy Thanksgiving. As you enjoy your dinner with your family, try to send some positive energy to me by osmosis. I'm hoping I'll be able to eat a Thanksgiving meal. They said I should be fine by Thursday, but I am going to take it slow. Talk to you after the surgery...

WEDNESDAY, NOVEMBER 25, 2009 4:41 PM; *48 days since my diagnosis.*

I'm out of surgery and at home. Still dealing with the anesthesia so my update will be short.

No drains!

FRIDAY, NOVEMBER 27, 2009 5:49 PM; *50 days since my diagnosis.*

Hello everyone. I hope you all had a great Thanksgiving day. I did. My brother and nephew came from Delaware to spend the holiday with me. We went over to my aunt's house where we had a great Thanksgiving Day meal. I was excited because I was able to eat my entire plate of food. Typically, anesthesia upsets my stomach.

I wanted to give you all an update on my surgery. As far as I know, everything went well. I arrived at the surgery center at 7:30 a.m. They called me to the back so I could get changed into my surgical outfit. I was draped nicely in a lavender gown accented with a deep purple bear paws. Did I mention the gown was heated? There were vent holes in the gown to allow for the heat to come in. The socks matched too. Once I was dressed for surgery, they put in an IV. Afterward, they called my family back to the area where I was. We sat in there for a while and then the doctor and physician assistant (PA) came to talk about the surgery.

Once the doctor and PA left, it was time for my mom and 'em to leave, too. Shortly after that, it was time for surgery. As I walked to the operating room, my nerves were beginning to get bad. I was very anxious. Once I got to the room and got up on the operating table, they put an EKG patch on my back. The nurse anesthetist told me she was giving me medicine through my IV and it might burn a little. They told me to lie back, and that was it. No counting backward. Nothing. The next thing I remember was them saying was, "You're all done."

I said, "Already? Do I have a drain?"

I guess that was the most important thing to me. I did not want a drain. As previously mentioned, having a drain would mean that I couldn't drive until it was taken out.

During surgery, I guess I talked a lot. The nurses told me I talked the entire time about my job and how I'm normally the one on the other side of the surgery room, working in a different capacity. Who would've thought I'd have a conversation under sedation? Especially one about work.

As I mentioned before, the surgeon performed a sentinel node biopsy. She injected dye into my breast tissue. The dye allowed the surgeon to see how the lymphatic fluid flowed so she could see which nodes would most likely have cancer cells. She removed the first lymph node (sentinel node) where the dye drained, and the next two additional ones. The were sent to be biopsied. Although, the results will not be available until next week, my surgeon thought she saw something while she was in there. She sent me to have another ultrasound. I was still groggy and feeling nauseous from the anesthesia. I experienced motion sickness as I was being wheeled through the hospital on a hospital bed.

Fortunately, the doctor who performed the ultra-

sound stated he didn't see anything. I was then released to go home. I didn't feel too good though. I was only able to eat crackers and drink ginger ale. I slept for most of the day. My cousin, Terri decided to stay with me that night. It was just like the good ole days when we were kids and we had sleepovers. We slept downstairs. I slept in the chair and she slept on the couch. My next appointment isn't until the end of next week. I will keep you all posted.

―――――――

[personal reflection]

Thinking back to this time period, I felt as though I was making some progress. Things were moving forward but still it felt as though I was in slow motion. I needed things to move at a faster pace. I was ready to start chemo and get this cancer out. Even though I knew it was not going to be easy, I was anxious to begin this battle. I was ready to be cancer-free again. I still had a long way to go but I was mentally prepared.

There were still so many unknowns. The results from the surgery were going to take a while to get, but I couldn't worry myself about that. I had to trust God and know that in all of this mess, there was a blessing to be found.

Reflection Questions

1. *What are you willing to do that scares you?*
2. *How will you mentally and physically prepare yourself?*
3. *Think of a time when you had to face adversity, do you recognize the blessing in it?*

7

it's worth a try, right?

"PART OF BEING OPTIMISTIC IS KEEPING ONE'S HEAD
POINTED TOWARD THE SUN, ONE'S FEET MOVING
FORWARD."

— NELSON MANDELA

This chapter of my book was not included in my
blog. Most people don't even know about this part of
my life. I had to ask myself if I should even share it.
The main purposes for me writing this book are to
both educate and inspire. I want people to be more

aware about breast cancer and all that's entailed with the battle. But more than anything, I want people to be inspired and know that if you have God in your life, you can accomplish things that you couldn't have imagined for yourself.

I'm not sure if this section will even be included in this book. If you're reading it, then you know that after much prayer, the Lord put it on my heart to share. Now you may ask, why are you writing this if you're not sure that you'll keep it the book? I think it's because I'm finding it therapeutic to write it down and revisit my feelings during this time. Writing this book has been very cathartic. This process was more emotional than I thought it would be. I am still amazed by how God has worked, and is still working in my life. I could not have made it through without Him. Anyway, here it goes...

As I was preparing to start my chemotherapy treatment, there were a lot of things going through my mind. Besides the fact I didn't want to die, I was 39 years old, single, with no children. Anyone who knows me, knows I love kids and the kids love me. I call myself the "child whisperer." Never did I think I would be that person who never had children.

After my cancer diagnosis, my best friend, Jackie kept begging me to go see a reproductive specialist to learn about my options. That was the furthest thing from my mind. I just wanted *life*. I wanted to beat this cancer thing and continue on living. However, since I was choosing to go through chemotherapy, the doctors didn't know how the chemotherapy drugs would affect my eggs. The doctor told me if I wanted to consider having children in the future, my best bet would be to either freeze my eggs or freeze embryos. I decided to begin the process.

There was a lot I didn't know about nonconventional fertility. The first step in the process was to meet with a reproductive endocrinologist. When I met with him, he explained the process. He went into details about egg freezing and embryo freezing. Egg freezing is just what it sounds like. It's when they take your eggs and freeze them. Believe it or not, egg freezing was still experimental at this time. Embryo freezing is when they take your egg, fertilize it, and then freeze it.

After our conversation about the In Vitro Fertilization (IVF) process, the doctor gave me a business card and told me to call the IVF nurses to find out what the next steps would be if I wanted to move forward with the process.

As soon as I arrived home, I called the IVF nurses to schedule a time to meet with them. I made an appointment to learn more about the process and a possible donor. I didn't know you could not use a known donor unless you were married or engaged to be married to that person. I had friends who offered their sperm and I truly appreciated them for that, but unfortunately I couldn't use them. I didn't completely understand the reasons behind why I couldn't use them, but I was told it was because of legal reasons. I tell you, I had never felt so vulnerable with my friends. Having those conversations had totally taken our friendships to another level.

In addition to scheduling appointments with the IVF nurses, I had to scheduled my appointments with the other members of reproductive team: the donor educator and social worker.

I only had a small window of time in which I could make all of this happen before chemo began. My oncologist was supportive of me going through the process, but not at the expense of me delaying my chemo treatment for more than two weeks.

Finally, I met with the reproductive team. It was a full day with a lot of information being shared. I went to the appointments with an open mind. I found out that the process would start once I began my menstrual cycle, which could be any day. Sorry if this is TMI. The team needed this to happen so that they could do a baseline assessment. The baseline assessment was necessary to ensure the ovaries are not producing eggs, test hormone levels, and make sure there are no cysts. Once my cycle started, the process would take about seven to ten days.

I was really anxious to meet with the donor educator. I was curious about the process of selecting a donor. The donor educator gave me two websites that I could use to select a donor. That's when I became stressed. *Am I really supposed to pick a 'baby daddy' from a website?* The only information the website gave me was the height, weight, eye color, hair color, ethnicity and profession...*if they had one.* I could pay extra money to get a baby picture of the donor if one was available. This was just too much.

Also, I had to meet with the social worker so that she could understand why I wanted to go through this process. She wanted to make sure my head was in the right place. I think I cried throughout the entire conversation. I still could not believe this was my life. Never did I think I would be at a fertility clinic talking about picking donors from a website.

I made daily appointments with the clinic in hopes that my menstrual cycle would start. Finally, after four days, it did. The timing was perfect. It would not delay my chemo treatment.

During my baseline appointment, the IVF nurses

were able to measure how many follicles I had. Each follicle had the potential to release an egg. While looking at my insides, the nurse said my ovaries were beautiful. What a nice compliment. LOL. Also, I had to get my blood drawn so that they could monitor my blood levels.

Going through the IVF process was very expensive. Besides the costs associated with the surgery to retrieve the eggs, the drugs cost thousands of dollars. I found out there are various organizations that focus specifically on helping breast cancer patients with fertility. The nurses gave me information regarding financial assistance that's available for breast cancer patients. Unfortunately, I didn't qualify for assistance, but I did have decent health insurance that helped with the surgery portion of it, but not with the drugs. The nurses were kind enough to give me some drugs that were donated from someone who didn't have to use all of theirs. For the rest of the drugs, I would have to pay out of pocket. It would all be worth it in the end.

On day three of my cycle, it was time for me to start my medications. I called the pharmacy to let them know I was on my way to pick up my medicine. The young lady, who answered the telephone, asked me for my medical ID number.

I replied, "M as in Mary, D as in David, C as in Cat, Z as in Z as in Zebra, X as in...Xylophone."

The young lady began to laugh. I asked her what was so funny and she responded, "X as in Xylophone."

It was in that moment I realized she probably thought xylophone started with a Z.

I asked, "What would you have said?"

She answered, "X as in ex-boyfriend."

Huh? I began to laugh. *Did she really say ex-boyfriend? She had to be joking, right? She could not be serious.* After a couple of seconds, I realized indeed she was serious. I just let it go.

Once I finished conversing with young lady, I had to call some of my close friends to share the story. It was hilarious to me. Each time I told it, I would crack myself up. I wasn't necessarily laughing at the young lady as much as I was the situation. I totally understood how she could've made the mistake. This story brought me some humor that I desperately needed in my life. Thank you young lady providing it for me.

When I finally went to pick up my medications, I made it a point to find that young lady. I needed to see who it was that didn't know the word ex-boyfriend started with an E and not a X. She was a very cute, petite young lady. She had medium length hair with highlights. I wanted to bring up our conversation to see if she seriously thought that ex-boyfriend started with a X, but I decided I would leave well enough alone. So instead, I just smiled.

When I was checking out, the pharmacist told me the price for some of my drugs. I realized just how expensive the drugs were. Yikes.

The first drug I had to take was Femara. This drug is used to help stimulate ovulation. This medication did not agree with me. It made me feel really crappy and made my heart race. I was scared to go to sleep that night because my heart was beating too fast. I was prescribed this medicine for four days, but I couldn't imagine having to take it another day. I questioned if I would be able to continue with the IVF process because I didn't think I would be able to deal with the side effects for three more days.

The next day, I told the nurse about my side effects. She said I could stop taking the Femara and start with the shots of Follistim. Thank goodness. Follistim was used to promote the growth and development of the eggs.

A little while later, the nurse called and told me I needed to be at the pharmacy by 5 p.m. to pick up the rest of my drugs. She said the drugs were free. *What? Did I hear her right? Did she say free?* Yes, she did. Look at God! This was further validation that He will make a way. I didn't really know the story behind how the nurses were able to get the medication at no cost to me. I had already bought some of the medication, but now I could pay it forward and donate the extra to someone else. I knew throughout this entire experience, God was with me. He had worked everything out. Praise God from whom all blessing flows...large and complex, small and simple.

The first time I had to give myself a shot of Follistim, it took me thirty minutes. I would poke my leg enough for it to start bleeding a little and then I would chicken out. After a while, the needle sort of slid into my skin. Afterward, I realized it wasn't bad at all. I guess just like chemo, the fear of the unknown had a grip on me. Each day, giving myself the shot became much easier.

After the fourth day of taking drugs, I had numerous eggs, but my estradiol level was low. This level is a measurement of the growth hormone for tissue of the reproductive organs. The nurses wanted to raise my estradiol level, so they had me increase my dosage of Follistim and start Ganirelix. This new drug was an antagonist which is primarily used to control ovulation. I had to continue to take both drugs for five more days.

I tell you, I was getting tired of this process. In addition to shooting myself with the drugs daily, my hormones were all over the place. I had mood swings, bloating, and hot flashes that would not stop. Fortunately, my estradiol levels increased and I had about nine to ten eggs, some with good size.

During this short amount of time, I had become very close with the IVF nurses. I guess it's because I had appointments with them every day, one for the ultrasound and one to get my blood drawn. The nurses were right there with me throughout the process. Besides being kind and compassionate, they were my biggest cheerleaders. They wanted me to succeed in the IVF process. They wanted me to have some viable eggs or embryos.

After nine days in this process, I had to inject myself with the final drug, the human chorionic gonadotropin (HCG). This drug was used to stimulate the release of the eggs. I had to mix together the solution and inject it at precisely 10:00 p.m. The drug injection had to be scheduled at that time because it needed to be exactly thirty-six hours before my surgery. There was no room for error with the time. This shot was the most painful because I had to inject medication into the muscle. I tried to do it on my own, but to no avail. Eventually, I had my friend help me. We tried to do the shot together, but I couldn't push the plunger. Eventually, I allowed him to shoot me in the leg.

The following day, my ovaries were huge. I felt as though my eggs were the size of golf balls. It was very uncomfortable. Fortunately, my surgery was schedule to take place at 10:00 a.m. the next day. Yay. I was almost at the finish line with this process.

Thirty-six hours after my last shot, I was finally able to have the surgery to retrieve my eggs. It has been a total of eleven days since my baseline assessment.

Jackie picked me up to take me to surgery. After we arrived at the hospital, the nurse called me back to go to the operating room area. They asked who I brought with me.

I answered, "My girlfriend, Jackie."

As the nurses walked out of the room, I saw them look back at me and then look to Jackie. I couldn't hear what they were saying, but something made me think they may have thought Jackie was my *girlfriend* for real. LOL.

A few minutes later, the nurse came in and had me sign the form so I could be enrolled as a study patient. As I mentioned before, egg freezing was still experimental at that time. Once the form was signed, I was all set to go to surgery.

The procedure to retrieve the eggs took about thirty minutes. Once it was over, I was sent back to recovery. I could hear people talking around me, but I wasn't quite ready to wake up yet.

I mumbled to Jackie, "What time is it?"

She told me that it was 11:00 a.m.

I told her, "Okay. I'll get up at 11:30 a.m. so we can leave."

Don't you know, at exactly 11:30 a.m., I *willed* myself to wake up.

I sat up and said, "I am ready to go."

Jackie laughed because, true to my word, I woke up at 11:30 a.m. on the dot. She always said once I put my mind to do something, I did it. I was determined because I was over being in the hospital.

I was happy I didn't have any nausea or pain after the procedure. I got up, got dressed, and then was pushed to the car in a wheelchair. I got in the car with Jackie and went to lunch. After we ate, Jackie took me back home. I was very tired. I rested for the remainder of the day. I did have some discomfort, but it wasn't anything Tylenol couldn't fix.

Later, I received a call from the doctor and he told me he was able to retrieve some viable eggs. "*Yes! All those shots were not in vain.*"

You may ask, "Was it worth it?" I would have to answer, "Yes." Going through this process gave me hope. My dream of having a child did not have to die because of my cancer diagnosis. There was still a possibility I could be a mother one day. If it was God's plan...

I am sharing this with you is because I didn't have anyone to share with me. I didn't know anyone who had gone through this process before and I didn't know what to expect. It would've been nice just to have someone to talk to and prepare me for what was to come. You may not know anyone who's going through IVF, but at least you have some knowledge of the process. Now back to the blog...

———

Reflection Questions

1. *What information are you willing to share that can help someone else in their journey?*
2. *What are you willing to risk to achieve your dreams and desires?*
3. *What steps can you take immediately that will lead you to those dreams and desires?*

8

facing giants

"KNOW YOUR ENEMY AND KNOW YOURSELF AND YOU
CAN FIGHT A HUNDRED BATTLES WITHOUT
DISASTER."

– SUN TZU

SUNDAY, NOVEMBER 29, 2009 8:49 AM; 52
days since my diagnosis.
D.O.B.: July 17th
Zodiac: Cancer
I WANT A NEW ZODIAC SIGN.

THURSDAY, DECEMBER 3, 2009 5:59 PM; 56 *days since my diagnosis.*

Well, today I met with the oncologist to get the results of the lymph node biopsy. They found the nodes were neither negative nor positive for cancer cells. "Huh?" I know I looked confused as they said this. From what I understood, there were a couple of cells in one node that were determined to be "in the middle." The initial testing found the cells to be negative, but now there's an additional way to do testing/ staining which was developed in the past five years. With this advanced testing, this was where the "middle-of-the-ground" cells were found. Nonetheless, my oncologist is suggesting that I do the less aggressive chemotherapy.

I won't have to start chemotherapy for a few a more weeks. Now I am able to go see the movie, The Princess and The Frog, when it comes out. Also, since I have some time before I start chemotherapy, they are going to do DNA testing on the cancer tumor. This will give them more information about the cancer and how it will/should respond to chemotherapy. I'll keep you all updated as we approach the target date.

FRIDAY, DECEMBER 4, 2009 4:12 PM; 57 days
since my diagnosis.

Okay, I misspoke yesterday. After seeing my surgeon today, I realized there was one "rare" cell out of
the two nodes, not two cells in one node. My surgeon
says this is good news. She asked about my appointment with the oncologist and wanted to make sure
I'm still doing chemotherapy to ensure that if any
cancer cells did get into my bloodstream, they will be
destroyed.

As for my post-op report from the lymph nodes
removal, there is a little fluid build-up underneath
my arm. That's where some of the tenderness I'm
experiencing is coming from. The doctor (and her
assistant) told me I should take it easy for a while (no
cleaning, etc.). I need to hire someone to do that for
me.

There is a light at the end of the tunnel though.
My doctor told me I should feel better in about eight
weeks. This is going to be a long-ish, slow journey.
I tell you, I didn't realize this surgery was like that.
I thought it was a "simple" procedure. However, the
doctor had to cut my nerves in order to remove the
lymph nodes. That is what's causing some of the
pain, too. The doctor told me my pain was going to

get worse before it gets better because the nerves have to regenerate themselves first. Also, it's important I continue to do my physical therapy on this arm, else it could lose its mobility.

Chemotherapy will begin soon. My date is tentatively set for December 21st. Once I complete my treatment, I'll have to go back and have the surgery to remove the remaining cancer tumor and some more lymph nodes to ensure the cancer still hadn't traveled.

THURSDAY, DECEMBER 10, 2009 6:40 PM; 63 *days since my diagnosis.*

I did get a bit of good news today. My genetic testing results came back and they were negative. The results showed I don't carry the genes for breast or ovarian cancer and therefore I will not have to have my ovaries removed. This will definitely have a positive impact on my next steps...well, the steps after chemotherapy.

WEDNESDAY, DECEMBER 16, 2009 10:20 PM; 69 *days since my diagnosis.*

I know it's been a few days since I've been on the blog. I've just been taking a mental break. This is the first week, in what seems like forever, that I didn't have a doctor's appointment. I am using this time to get my psyche right before I start chemotherapy. It still seems surreal to me at times.

Yesterday, I went to the "Look Good...Feel Better" workshop that was sponsored by the American Cancer Society. There are many changes in appearances that one goes through during chemotherapy and this class gave helpful hints on how to look good, which in turn will make one feel better. When I arrived, I received a bag with various skin care items as well as cosmetics. All the cosmetics were donated to the organization. I received some Mary Kay cleanser; Chanel, Mac Cosmetics, and Bobbi Brown make-up; and a whole lot of other goodies. The bag and its contents have to be worth about $200. As a make-up junkie, I was very excited. Anyone who knows me knows I love to play with make-up.

The "Look Good...Feel Better" workshop also dealt with the most noticeable change one experiences when going through chemo, hair loss. They demonstrated how to use wigs, turbans and scarves as a way to cover the head after hair loss. Besides the workshop being informative, it was free.

I was the only person in the class who hadn't started treatment yet, but it was good seeing others doing well as they went through their treatment. Some had already lost their hair and some were in the process of losing their hair. It's amazing how much hair matters to women.

Surprisingly, there were people going through chemo who hadn't even shared it with anyone besides their spouses. Not their children, not other family members, not their best friends, no one. I understand everyone isn't like me, but selfishly, I needed people to know about my situation. One, because I needed their prayers for healing, strength, and even quiet moments. Secondly, for awareness about breast cancer.

Another nice thing about the workshop is it gave those people who hadn't shared their journey an opportunity to talk about the situation with others who are going through it.

Before I finish blogging, I want to leave you with the following scripture that was in a card that I received.

"I will not leave you comfortless: I will come to you." – John 14:18 (KJV)

What a great reminder to know I'm not alone. During my quiet moments, I can feel God's presence with

me. I praise Him for being my Comforter and for giving me the endurance to keep pressing.

WEDNESDAY, DECEMBER 16, 2009 10:52 PM;
69 days since my diagnosis; 32 minutes since my last
post.

Okay, I'm back again...briefly. I forgot to mention in the last journal update that I received a butterfly figurine from the "Look Good...Feel Better"
workshop. The figurine consists of a beautiful, fiery
orange butterfly which is perched on a branch. The
inscription on the base of the stand reads, "Just when
the caterpillar thought the world was over, it became
a butterfly." Sheri's Butterfly (that's the name) is
given as a special symbol of personal inspiration and
determination. Just like the caterpillar, I will be
transformed. I am excited to experience my transformation and see the person I become.

———————

[personal reflection]

I had been going through the motions, living somewhat in a state of shock. I was tired of cancer already.
It sucked! Did I say I was tired of cancer already?
This was getting old and the difficult part was that
the major battle hadn't even begun. When I think

back to this time, I must admit I was a little scared. Defeating cancer wasn't going to be easy. It was not going to be a quick, one-two combo punch; it was going to take many rounds to get that knockout.

When people hear the word *cancer*, they automatically think of suffering, dying and/or death. That little six-letter word can hold a lot of power. In order to defeat it, I couldn't give cancer any power over my life. I was tired of hearing the word cancer and especially tired of it being in my body. I looked forward to the days of being cancer-free again, but first I had to confront and defeat the giant in my life – cancer.

I was reminded of the story of David and Goliath. Just like David, we all will face "giants" in our lives. We all will have "giant" problems and seemingly impossible situations we will have to go up against. Giants are anything that can distract us from focusing on God. There's the giant called *depression*. The giant called *worry*. The giant called *fear*. The giant called *doubt*. There's even a giant called *payment due*, which you may face when you don't have enough money to pay your bills. I could go on and on listing the many "giants" that exist, but you get the point.

In the story, there are many lessons to be learned

about facing giants. I'm not a pastor, so I'm not going to give a full sermon on the text. However, I will touch briefly on some of the points that stood out for me in the story.

David lets us know he was very disappointed with the Israelites because they were too afraid to stand up against Goliath, even though he defied the army of God. He became fed up and couldn't take the insults and mockery anymore. Having been overlooked, David decided to step up and take action.

He went before Saul and said to him, "Let no one lose heart on account of this Philistine; your servant will go and fight him."

Saul told David he wasn't ready to fight him. "You are only a young man, and he (Goliath) has been a warrior from his youth."

David replied, "Your servant has been keeping his father's sheep. When a lion or a bear came and carried off a sheep from the flock, I went after it, struck it and rescued the sheep from its mouth. When it turned on me, I seized it by its hair, struck it and killed it."

David was letting Saul know he was already prepared for the battle with the Philistine. Just like David, we too are prepared when giants arise in our lives. Even though we may not believe it, all the tests and trials that we've experienced in our lives have prepared us to be victorious against any challenge that comes our way.

Secondly, David was just a young boy who had gone to check on his brothers at the request of his father. While he was there, he became curious as to why the Israelites feared Goliath and allowed him to mock them. Everyone was afraid to take Goliath up on his offer to fight—everyone except David. He didn't allow his beliefs to conform to those of the others. David had his confidence in God and trusted that Goliath could be defeated.

"With man this is impossible, but with God all things are possible." – Matthew 19:26 (NIV)

David had the vision of a giraffe. I know this statement came out of left field but do you understand what I'm talking about when I say that? Let me explain.

Bishop T.D. Jakes, who is the founder and senior pastor of The Potter's House, in Dallas, TX, spoke to this. He has written a book, *Instinct: The Power to Unleash Your Inborn Drive*, where he talks about why some people are unable to share in your vision. These people are the naysayers in your life. Most of us have dealt with them at some point. They are the people who try to tell you what you can't do instead of what you can. You've heard them before. "That won't work. You can't do that. You aren't smart enough. You're too short to play in the NBA. You're too tall to be a ballerina." You get the point. These are the people who try to discourage you at every turn.

I will do my best to paraphrase my interpretation of what Bishop T.D. Jakes says about dealing with the naysayers. I may not describe it as eloquently as he does, but I'll give it a try. My apologies in advance to you Bishop T.D. Jakes...just in case you're reading this.

Bishop T.D. Jakes talks about the differences between turtles and giraffes. Giraffes are mainly known for their tall stature, long neck, and long legs. Conversely, turtles have short, sturdy limbs and are low to the ground. Even though giraffes and turtles may occupy the same space, their perspectives are from different vantage points. A turtle has a limited view because it can only see from its level, whereas the giraffe has a higher, broader view. So when naysayers say *you can't*, it's only because they can't see what *you can* from their vantage point. "Just 'cause you can't see it don't mean it ain't." I know that's bad language and I just made that up...I think.

Giraffes are designed to be tall. They eat from

trees. If they tried to eat off of the ground with a turtle, it would strangle itself. The giraffe will endanger its position when it tries to lower its perspective.

Applying this to the story of David and Goliath, David was a giraffe. David's faith in God caused him to look at the giant from a different perspective than the other Israelites (the naysayers a.k.a. turtles). The Israelites believed the giant couldn't be defeated, but David looked at Goliath as merely a mortal man who defied God. Rather than having a turtle's perspective and believing in defeat, David aligned his perspective with the higher, broader view. God's point of view. Because of that, David was able to annihilate Goliath.

The last point I am going to make is that David was not afraid to face the giant. The scripture says, "As the Philistine moved closer to the attack him, David ran quickly toward the battle line to meet him." While everyone else allowed Goliath to paralyze them, David ran toward the giant. This is a reminder that we must confront our giants head on. We must go confidently and courageously in the direction of our challenge. If you have fear, you must feel the fear, but do it anyway. Your trust has to be in the Lord. You can't have one hand pulling you toward FAITH and the other viciously pulling you towards FEAR. That will keep you stuck in place. Paralyzed. Without any movement. Without any action. Faith and fear cannot co-exist in the same space. You have to make a decision. Either you focus on God and trust Him, or you give in to fear and become defeated. The choice is yours.

My giant happened to be called cancer. It would've be easy to wave my white flag and assume the position of 'man down', but I know I couldn't. I didn't want to be defeated. When I looked at my "giant" from God's perspective, I realized God would fight for me and with me. I had to trust God and give it over to Him. This battle wasn't mine; it was the Lord's. (II Chronicles 20:15) The bible says, "Cast all your anxiety on him because he cares for you." – 1 Peter 5:7 (NIV)

That is exactly what I did. I put my confidence in God and believed that everything was going to be alright. Now am I saying I didn't have to do any work? *No, not at all.* What I am saying is that I was willing to do my part and trusted God would do His. Even though I may not have understood why this was my life, I continued to stand on His promises.

I remember talking to a friend about my situation and he asked me, "Do ever you wonder why God would allow this to happen to you? You're such a good person."

I replied, "No, I've never waste my energy on the 'why me.' I always take the approach, 'why not me?' The fact of the matter is that it was what it was. There's nothing I can do about my situation. I had cancer. However, I know everything happens for a reason. I may not understand it, but I trust it. I consider myself a strong and resilient person and I know I will get through this."

Did I think the battle would be easy? *No.* Would I fight with all my might? *Yes.* I know for a fact giants do die. David showed us that. The bigger they are, the harder they fall. Bring on chemo. I was ready...

———

Reflection Questions

1. *What is the giant in your life?*
2. *What weapons to do you need to annihilate it?*
3. *What steps can you take to right now to defeat it?*

9

chemo, chemo take it away!

"IF YOU COULD GET UP THE COURAGE TO BEGIN, YOU
HAVE THE COURAGE TO SUCCEED."

– DAVID VISCOTT

MONDAY, DECEMBER 21, 2009 8:05 AM; 74
days since my diagnosis.

*Today is the day! My first chemotherapy treat-
ment will start soon. I'm not sure how I thought I'd*

feel this morning, but right now I'm okay. I had a decent night of sleep and now I'm just waiting to be picked up by my mom and Jackie so they can take me to my appointment. I'll probably get a little emotional once they start the treatment. I pray that I get through it fine. Please keep me in prayer. My appointment with my oncologist is a 9:00 a.m. and my treatment begins at 9:30 a.m.

MONDAY, DECEMBER 21, 2009 11:18 PM; 74 *days since my diagnosis...after my first chemo treatment.*

It's Monday night at 11:18 p.m., and I have not gone to sleep yet. I have been sooooo tired all day, but I can't seem to fall asleep. I'm hoping that once I take a warm bath and get between my flannel sheets, things will change quickly. I figured since I'm wide awake, I'd share how my day went.

When I arrived for my appointment, I met with my oncologist. He asked me how I was doing and if I was ready to start treatment. I reiterated that I didn't understand why I had to start chemo right before Christmas. I thought next week would've been a better time to start. Matter of fact, why not wait until after the new year? Can you believe I'm saying *that? Initially, all I wanted was to start treatment. Now, I wanted to delay it and wait until after the holidays. My doctor believed that I'd do fine with the treatment so changing the day wasn't even up for discussion. However, what was up for discussion was if I wanted to do chemotherapy at all. He told me he received my DNA results on the cancer and my number came back low. I guess you want to know what that means, huh? So did I. The range of the score can be anywhere from zero to one hundred. Mine was fifteen. Women with lower scores have a lower risk that their cancer will return. These women also have a cancer that is less likely to respond to chemo.*

Here I was, five minutes away from beginning my first chemo treatment and my oncologist is asking me if I even wanted to do this. I asked him to give me a moment with my mom and Jackie so we could discuss in private. Can you believe this? It has taken me one and one-half months to get my mind psyched for chemotherapy and now he's saying I will only get minimal benefits from it. *Sigh* Minimal or not, I feel there are some benefits from doing chemotherapy. If you remember from my previous surgery, there was a "rare" cell that was found in one of the nodes. We don't know much about that rare cell, but I would feel better knowing I'm treating my whole body just in case a cancer cell was able to travel to another location. Secondly, chemotherapy will help reduce the size of the tumor and it would help in the preservation of my breast and minimize deformity, if I decide to do a lumpectomy.

During the five minutes we were given to discuss whether I would do chemo or not, Jackie and my mom talked while I went to the restroom. My mind was already made up, however, I did value their opinion. They know me best and know I would drive myself insane if I didn't go through this process. I wanted to do all I could do to ensure that I didn't hear the words "YOU HAVE BREAST CANCER" again. Any minimal benefit is worth it to me.

Needless to say, I started my treatment today; I received the less aggressive drug therapy at a low dose. My main side effects will be fatigue and hair loss. Also, I will have to be careful about being around people who are sick because of the possibility of infection is increased with my low immune system.

Anyway, I was put into my private room about 10 a.m. They put an IV in my arm and then mixed up the drugs I had to receive. The nurses were not allowed to prepare the medications until it was *about to be used. Also, it was a requirement that three people sign off on each medication and dosage. The hospital protects the patients (and itself) by triple checking to ensure they are dispensing the correct drugs and the correct dosage.*

I became very nervous. My legs just kept shaking and I kept having to use the restroom. In the few hours I was there, I think I went to the restroom about ten times. I found myself going to the restroom every time they checked my blood pressure or changed the medications.

The first IV drug I was given was Pepcid (I guess to control indigestion). Next, I was given an IV steroid, the same steroid I had to take last night and earlier this morning. The nurse mentioned that this drug will probably keep me awake, even when I feel tired. Go figure. It took about fifteen minutes to get the steroid into my system.

Next, it was time for the chemotherapy agents. My legs were really shaking at this point. The first chemotherapy agent I received was Taxotere. This drug was supposed to take no more than an hour to run through the IV. Unfortunately, within the first fifteen minutes, I had a reaction. My arm became unusually hot. The doctor came in and slowed the

IV drip for a while. After things calmed down, he sped the drip back up over time. That seemed to work better. It took about one and one-half to two hours to get all of the drug into my system. The next drug I received was Cytoxan. This was only supposed to take forty-five minutes to an hour, but it took much longer. By the time it was all over, my two-hour session ended up taking almost four hours.

Even though there were some glitches, I was comfortable with taking this "optional" chemotherapy treatment. I know me and I know I would have regrets if I didn't do the treatment. I need to have a free conscience and feel as though I'm giving it my all. My life is at stake. I don't know what God has in store for me, but I do know I have to go through the process and live out His plan. I will do it to the best of my ability.

Emotionally, it wasn't that bad going through the treatment. Yes, I was nervous, but it was nice to have distractions with other people being there. My mom, Jackie, and other family members and friends came and sat with me. We talked about remodeling Jackie's kitchen, watched The Wendy William's Show ("How You Doin'?") and watched The View. Unfortunately, no one wanted to watch my favorite movie, *Die Hard*. I really wanted to see Bruce Willis kick butt again. Even though I had seen the movie one hundred ninety-nine times, I thought it was an appropriate movie to watch because the movie took place around Christmas time and it's the Christmas season. Yippie Ki Yay...

I will be back blogging tomorrow to let you know how things go for me tonight. Also, I'll update you on my next appointment scheduled for tomorrow afternoon. I have to get a shot to help build up my white blood cells. I hope you resting well and that I will be joining you soon.

WEDNESDAY, DECEMBER 23, 2009 9:19 AM; 76 days since my diagnosis.

I apologize that I didn't get a chance to blog yesterday. After waking up yesterday morning, I noticed issues with my right eye. I kept seeing floaters that were hindering my vision. Around 10:00 a.m., my nurse called to ask me how I was feeling and if I'd noticed anything different. I told her about the floaters and she told me to stop taking my anti-nausea medication since it makes me drowsy and I may have to drive to the eye doctor.

First, I went to my doctor's office to get my follow-

up shot which helps boost my white blood cells. After the shot, I had to go to the emergency eye center to see the eye doctor. I had my mom drive me to the eye appointment because I was told I may need to have my pupils dilated.

After I arrived to the emergency eye center, I had my examination. My vision was 20/20 in both eyes. The ophthalmologist told me he wants me to meet with an eye cancer specialist. Eye cancer specialist?!? I couldn't believe what he was saying. It reminded me of the lady I met at The Gathering Place who was diagnosed with breast cancer after it presented itself in her eye. Can my life get any worse right now? Can some things please just be routine for a change?

Anyway, the eye cancer specialist shot dye into my eye so he could see my blood vessels and determine where the blockage was occurring. Fortunately, he didn't see anything. No blockage, nor tumor. That was great news, however there was something going on that was causing the floaters and creating a blockage. I was scheduled for another appointment in three weeks. Meanwhile, the specialist said the floaters should go away eventually. I'm hoping he is correct because this big, grey floater is really hindering my vision.

Once the eye exam was finished, I went home and tried to nap. I was still having a difficult time falling asleep. Later in the day, Jackie and my Raggedies (Aaliyah, India and Erin), came by to bring me some of white chocolate cranberry cookies from the mall. Yummy. My Raggedies are Jackie's daughters and my goddaughters. Aaliyah Janae is 7 years old. India Andrea and Erin Yvonne are 5-year old twins. I affectionately call them my Raggedies because uhh well, umm, because...did I say how great they are? Well, they are. LOL. But seriously, they are great girls who also just happen to be very intelligent and perceptive.

My cousins, Terri and Teryn stopped by, too. I had a house full. I went upstairs to show off the wigs I bought to cover my head when my hair falls out. I bought three different wigs for different occasions and different moods. One of the wigs was a dark brown, bob cut that I could wear to work. The second one was an asymmetrical, medium brown colored wig that looked like a hairstyle that I had worn many years ago. The final wig was my favorite because it was a style I had never worn before. It was a long, laced-front, straight wig with a part down the middle. Never, and I mean never, have I had long hair. I don't even really like myself with much hair, but I thought this wig would tap into another personality that has been bottled up inside of me.

When I brought the wigs downstairs, I modeled each one of them. Aaliyah, my oldest Raggedy, asked me why was I trying on wigs. I told her I was doing it just in case my hair fell out.

Then she asked, "Do you have cancer?"

I was totally caught off guard. I hadn't shared with the Raggedies anything about my situation because they were so young. Sadly, I responded, "Yes." I asked how did she know about cancer and she said that she remembered seeing the little girl without hair on TV and she had cancer. Then she told me, "I don't want you to die."

Those words broke my heart. I told her I wasn't going to die. She looked at me and then asked if she could cry into my pillow on the couch.

I'm still crying thinking about the look on her face. She looked so sad and scared. With this, I am going to end this blog for today since I can barely see with all the tears...and floaters.

SUNDAY, DECEMBER 27, 2009 8:42 PM; 80 days
since my diagnosis.

Okay, here we are on Sunday evening, almost
one week since my first treatment. This has been a
little more difficult than I expected. Not because of
the chemotherapy, I feel as though I tolerated that
well. There were a few of days where my stomach
wasn't settled and I could taste the chemo. It was
a horrible, metallic taste. Yuck. However, my main
problem is the bone pain which was a result of the
shot I received the day after my chemotherapy treatment. That shot has had me in pain since Wednesday night. It's almost unbearable. I have been lying
in the fetal position all day. This bone pain is intense.
It hurts to even walk on the soles of my feet. The
pain feels as though someone is squeezing my bones/
skull with vice grips. Terrible, terrible, terrible, excruciating pain. I've been taking some pain meds which
have helped a little. I am going to keep on pressing
on and keep reminding myself this is only temporary.
Only for a moment. That is how I have to psyche
myself out. I've called the doctor numerous times
about this and he said it should last only one to two
days. I am now on day four. I pray the pain will subside soon.

In addition to the pain, my back is itching and feels like it's on fire. When I scratch my back, it feels as though I am scratching off my skin. Even though I know I'm really not scratching off my skin, I still check under my fingernails to see if there is any skin. Nothing. At some point, I decided to look at my back in the mirror. To my surprise, I saw a burn. What in the world? Where did this come from? The burn is the size of a nickel. It is just something else I had to deal with. I am a miserable mess.

I'm also dealing with other side effects. For the past couple of nights, I've been experiencing a fast heart rate. My heart feels like it going to jump out of my chest. Also, I've noticed I've been having some issues with my memory. It's been difficult remembering some things. It's very frustrating.

Even though it's the holiday weekend, I called the oncologist's office to let them know about all the side effects I was experiencing: the bone pain, burn on my back, rapid heart rate, and memory issues. I needed some answers as to what I could do to help resolve these problems. I spoke to the nurse and she told me the pain should be able to be controlled by ibuprofen or Vicodin. She also mentioned that the memory loss is probably from the anxiety medication. They are not sure about the burn or fast heart rates. They are going to tweak my medications the next time I receive chemo to help reduce or possibly eliminate the side effects.

I have an appointment for an MRI tomorrow. After the eye exam last week for the floater, the doctor just wants to make sure everything is okay with my head (no jokes, please). Hopefully, the bad weather that's supposed to come will wait until after 5 p.m. A winter storm can paralyze the city. Did I say how much I very much dislike the winters in Cleveland? Well, I do.

TUESDAY, DECEMBER 29, 2009 9:46 AM; 82 *days since my diagnosis.*

GOOD NEWS!!! I just received a call from the eye doctor and my MRI from yesterday was fine. He didn't see anything on the images. Now, I just have to wait for the blockage of the blood vessel in my eye to heal itself and then the floaters should be gone. My eyesight is definitely getting better each day.

New Side Effect Alert: My fingertips are hurting. It feels like a million pins are sticking them. I called the doctor's office and the nurse said my nerve endings are probably damaged from the chemo. They want me to keep an eye on it. There's nothing that can be done about it except to wait it out. Unfortunately, the side effects from the chemo drugs are cumulative, meaning that after the next treatment, I may have the issues with my fingertips again, but next time it would be sooner and/or longer in duration.

FRIDAY, JANUARY 1, 2010 10:57 PM; 85 *days since my diagnosis.*

Happy New Year's Day to you all! I am praying that you (and me) have a HEALTHY, prosperous and blessed year in 2010.

Today, was a good day. I used this day to relax and reflect on what's to come. My life totally changed three months ago. I would've never thought on January 1, 2010, I would be in the battle for my life. But here I am, by the grace of God, starting a new year with a new perspective and new attitude. I know in all of this mess, there's a blessing to be found (I just love saying that). I'm able to confront my illness and know that no matter what, this experience is for my good.

Last night, I went to my church's watchnight service where I ministered with the choir. I thank God for giving me the strength to be able to do that. I was not sure if I was going to make it, or even if I should. However, my doctor thought I was well enough to go to church. I didn't stay long, though, because there were several people all around me coughing and blowing their noses. I cannot allow myself to get sick. My immune system isn't strong enough yet. Before I left, one of our former choir members sang the song "Safe in His Arms" by Rev. Milton Brunson. We used to sing this song years ago, but it was just what I needed to hear last night. If you're not familiar with the song, the lyrics are as follows:

> *Because the Lord is my shepherd,*
> *I have everything I need.*
> *He lets me rest in the meadow's grass*
> *and He leads me beside the quiet streams,*
> **He restoreth my failing health,**
> *and He helps me to do what*
> *honors Him the most;*
> *that's why I'm safe, that's why I'm safe,*
> *that's why I'm safe, safe in His arms.* [2]

Although I already know it, it's great reassurance to hear that I am safe in His arms. He is my Protector.

On a side note, I still have hair. I am not sure if

I'll lose it or not, but if I do, most likely it'll happen sometime soon.

Oh, I have another story from my 7-year-old Raggedy, Aaliyah. As you may recall, she was the one who asked if I had cancer when I was trying on wigs a couple of weeks ago. Evidently, my situation is really bothering her. Yesterday, she kept bringing it up to me. She asked if I still had cancer. Why did I have to have cancer? Am I upset about having cancer?

In order to ease her mind, I reassured her that I'll be fine. It's difficult knowing how much this is affecting her. I wanted to cry, but I couldn't in front of her. It would make her sadder and more anxious. Anyway, as she sat watching TV, a commercial for Bosley Hair Restoration came on.

I was in the kitchen at the time and Aaliyah ran into the room, pointing at the TV and said, "Auntie Andrea, you don't have to wear your wigs. You can get that!" She was so excited I didn't have to be bald and that Bosley could solve my hair loss issues. I tell you, children say the darnedest things. It was very sweet knowing that she loves me and she's trying to help fix my problems.

Since Aaliyah was having a difficult time with

my situation, Jackie suggested maybe we not use the word "chemo" anymore. Instead, she said we should call it "K."

I asked her why K?

She said, "K for kemo."

I busted out laughing. "Umm, Jackie, chemo doesn't begin with the letter K."

This is reminiscent of the young lady at the pharmacy who said "X" is for ex-boyfriend. LOL.

Anyway, I will keep you posted with my progress. As I mentioned before, I am doing okay. There are a lot of side effects I wasn't prepared for, but I am learning more and more about my strength every day. I can't wait to see how God is going to use me after all of this.

Love, peace, and blessings to all. Remember to be grateful for life and all it has to offer. Be sure to treasure the precious moments with family and loved ones and not take them for granted.

New Side Effect Alert: My toes are tingling and my fingernails are starting to turn dark around the cuticles. I started painting my nails with dark polish.

———

[personal reflection]

The fear of the unknown is what made chemo scary. I didn't know what to expect. Although I was prepped with what *could* happened while going through chemo, I know that everyone reacts differently. At this point, I had experienced some yucky side effects already. However, I knew this was what I had to go through to get me to my goal of being cancer-free.

I was grateful for my life...even with cancer. This definitely wasn't how I would have designed it, however there was a gift to be found going through this. There was a blessing on the other side waiting for me to receive it. Because of that, I made a conscious decision to continue to fight and have an attitude of gratitude.

Reflection Questions

1. *What are you grateful for?*
2. *How can you incorporate gratitude in your life?*
3. *What steps do you need to take in order to be more appreciative of the curve balls that life throws your way?*

10

my bald is beautiful

"BEAUTY IS NOT CAUSED. IT IS."

— EMILY DICKINSON

———

THURSDAY, JANUARY 7, 2010 5:16 PM; 91 *days*
since my diagnosis.

Adios...

Au Revoir...

Caio...

Auf Wiedersehen...

GOODBYE HAIR...

... *you will be missed while you're gone.*

Well, it seems like the inevitable is now happening. My hair has been falling out since Sunday. Today, I can see where there are patches of missing hair. I've tried to cover it up as much as possible, but I guess it's time for me to make the decision whether or not I should shave the rest or just continue to let it come out in clumps. Decisions, decisions, decisions. I'm not really ready to lose my hair. Although I know that my hair loss is temporary, it's still a loss.

Before I finish blogging, I want to thank one of the deaconesses from my church who mentioned she will shave her head in support of my situation. I must say it's so not necessary. It's cold outside. Unfortunately, I don't have a choice in this hair loss battle, but she does. You know who you are. Please keep your hair.

I am now preparing for my second round of chemotherapy. After that one, I'll be half-way there...at least with the chemo. There is a light...

THURSDAY, JANUARY 7, 2010 11:28 PM; 91 days *since my diagnosis; 6 hours and 12 minutes since my last post.*

Surprisingly, tonight wasn't emotional for me. As an update to my earlier post, my hair is now gone. I could have continued to let it fall out at its leisure, but I decided to take things into my own hands and to shave it off completely.

Wait, let me back up a little. I didn't know what I was going to do with my hair once it began to come out. However, my girlfriend, Nakia called after she read my earlier blog. She asked me if I wanted her to cut it off.

After giving some thought to the idea about cutting off my hair, I said, "Why not? Let's just get this over with."

She drove over through all of the snow to come and chop off the little hair I had left. That is so Nakia. She has always been that person who does whatever she can to make someone feel better. She and I met some years ago when I was assigned to be her prayer partner at church and we have been close friends ever since.

As she started cutting my hair, the first look we went for was the Mohawk look. She shaved the sides and kept the top longer. Just as we finished cutting my hair into a mohawk, Jackie arrived. She had called me earlier to see how I was doing. I told her that I was going to cut off my hair, so she came over to check on me and make sure that I was okay.

Nakia continued to cut off my remaining hair. I

looked a mess because there were some areas that we couldn't cut close enough to my scalp. Fortunately, I had some other clippers that was able to cut closer. I decided to participate in the final stage of cutting of my hair. Surprisingly, it was liberating to be a part of the experience.

After my hair was completely shaved off, my scalp was washed, conditioned and moisturized with shea butter. Wait a minute, I got this all wrong. I got my hair washed, conditioned and moisturized before I cut my hair with the second pair of clippers. It was while I was drying my hair with the towel that I realized that some hair was still coming out. That's when I went to get the other clippers to cut it off completely. After we finished, I threw my hair into the garbage can. All of a sudden, Jackie says, "Let's have a hair burning ceremony."

My initial thought was, "What in the world is a hair burning ceremony?" Jackie didn't want me to just throw my hair away with the garbage; she wanted me to memorialize it. I told her I was a little leery because I didn't want my house to burn down participating this "made up" ceremony.

Jackie said, "Well let's go outside. The house won't catch on fire if we do it outside."

I thought about it for a quick moment then realized it was just too cold outside, plus my neighbors might think we were crazy.

Nakia asked, "Jackie, how should we do this? You're the firefighter's wife!"

Being true to her role, Jackie suggested we put some aluminum foil in the sink and burn it.

I got some matches and attempted to set the hair on fire. However, before I got a chance to light it, Jackie said, "You have to say something first."

"What am I supposed to say to my hair?" I had no idea as to what to say. I told my hair that I enjoyed it being a part of my life for the last 39 years and that I couldn't wait 'til we meet again. LOL.

As the hair burned in the sink, we joked about how weird the burning hair looked and the fact that there wasn't any smell nor smoke. Then all of a sudden, my smoke detector in the kitchen started going off. I ran to open the door and fan the area. Even though we didn't see the smoke, there must've been some.

Once we were able to get the kitchen smoke detector to stop beeping, my basement's smoke detector went off. How did that happen? Evidently, the invisible smoke traveled down there, too. We laughed *so hard that tears were rolling down our faces. This incident brought us back to the realization that this was a silly thing to do in the first place. However, thank you Jackie for giving us this idea...and a good laugh.*

After the ceremony, we took pictures of my bald head. I realized how much I look like my daddy. Wow.

I tried on my wigs again and some headscarves. Now that I'm bald, I need to decide which look I want to have. I am not the one to walk around with a bald head. Plus, I have to make sure that my head stays warm.

[personal reflection]

After I posted about losing my hair, my friend, Nichelle sent me a message. "YOU ARE NOT YOUR HAIR." She was right. I didn't need to stress over the fact I didn't have hair anymore or even care about what others might think. My hair didn't define who I was. I was more than my hair. I was still beautiful.

Reflection Questions

1. *Where do you find beauty in your life?*
2. *How can you be intentional about recognizing the beauty in all things?*
3. *What silly thing have you done that made you laugh until you cried?*

11

chemo: round two

"ONLY THOSE WHO WILL RISK GOING TOO FAR CAN
POSSIBLY FIND OUT HOW FAR ONE CAN GO."

– T. S. ELIOT

MONDAY, JANUARY 11, 2010 11:28 PM; *95 days
since my diagnosis.*

*Chemotherapy Treatment Number Two: Last
night, I didn't fall asleep until 3:00 a.m. I think I
was subconsciously anticipating my treatment. I was
back up at 7:00 a.m. waiting for my noon appoint-*

ment. After I arrived at the clinic, I met with my nurse and oncologist. I shared with them all of the side effects that I experienced over these past three weeks. They were shocked I had experienced all of the ones that were expected and more. Their main concern was the remaining floater in my eye. They don't believe it's from the chemotherapy agents, but instead from the changes in my estrogen levels. I have another appointment with the eye doctor tomorrow morning and hopefully I'll get some more information. Their other concern was the excruciating bone pain I had to endure for the seven to eight days after the last chemo treatment. That was the worst.

Initially, the doctor didn't know how to manage the pain. After a few days of experiencing the bone pain, the doctor finally prescribed me some drugs that actually made the pain more manageable. However, when the bone pain began to subside, my joints began to ache. Then after the joint aches left, I started getting horrible headaches. It seemed like a never ending cycle. However, after one and one-half weeks, the pain was gone for good.

I wasn't sure which drug caused the pain after the treatment, but I knew if they couldn't figure it out, I wasn't doing another chemotherapy treatment.

Jackie kept trying to convince me I would regret not completing all of the treatments. But as bad as the pain was, I did not care if I stopped at that point. It was horrible and I couldn't sleep.

However, I found out after just one treatment, the chemotherapy seems to be working. My oncologist said that the tumor is shrinking and it's about half the size that it was before I started. That was good news. Even better news, I don't have to take the shot the day after my chemotherapy treatment again. My oncologist believes it was the cause of my pain. One of the chemotherapy agents I still have to take can cause me to feel achy, but hopefully the pain won't be as intense as the last time. We will see how it goes.

The shot that I don't have to take anymore is the one that helps boost my white blood cell levels. I would rather just stay away from people to protect my immune system instead of getting that shot again. I have a 10 percent chance of catching an infection and worst case scenario is that I'll end up in the hospital for three to four days. I know what you're thinking, "Is it worth taking that risk?" My answer is "Yes." I had never, ever, ever felt pain like that before. It was a constant, excruciating pain that would subside for only about five minutes and then come back with a vengeance. I was living in a zombie state during that time. My family and friends felt so bad for me when they saw me in such pain.

I pray this time is going to be much better since I'm refusing the shot. The only thing that will be different is I have to get my blood tested in eight days to make sure my white blood count is increasing like it should.

When they took my blood pressure, it was pretty good. I was surprised because it was a little elevated the last time I received treatment. They took my blood to check the levels to see if they needed to modify anything.

As far as the process, it was the same as the last time. I took my two Benadryls, IV of Pepcid, Zofran, Dexamethasone, and then my two chemotherapy agents, Taxotere and Cytoxan. It took a little less than four hours to receive all the drugs.

I decided to wear the same outfit from when I had my first treatment. It makes it easier to go to the restroom since I have to go frequently while I'm getting my treatment. This time I wore my rosary beads because they match perfectly with my outfit. Also, I wore a matching headscarf to cover my bald head.

I am tired, but I wanted to get this blog out

tonight because one of the drugs I'm on gives me short-term memory loss. By tomorrow, I may very well forget what happened today.

TUESDAY, JANUARY 12, 2010 10:36 AM; 96 days since my diagnosis.

I thought it would be fun to try to type this journal update nafter having my eyes dialated. I can't haredly see a thing so I I know there is going to be many typos. Hipefully, you all will be able to follow me. As an aside, I may edit this once myvision comes back completely. Any, I had my follow-up eye exam this morning. It pretty mch confirmed what I had already knew. The eye doctor seems to think that one of the chemo agents that I'm taking is the cause of the blockkage (or clt) in my vessel. They just want to continue to monitor the eye and see if there's any changes. So far, they don't think that I have need to worry. My age plays a factor in it's healing and they think I should be bind. I won' have to go back until March 15th. That will be after my last chemo treatment and hopefully my eye will be on the road to recovery. WEll, that's it for now. I must get off this computer because I literally can't see anything and I'm just typing away and sometimes can't see if I'm *typing workds twices. I do know that there are some misspelled words, but I can't tell which ones. I'm hoping after the nap I am able to take, I'll be be able to see again. Take care care. I just just wnated to getve you challenge of hte day. Try to figrue out what I was tryng to say.*

SUNDAY, JANUARY 17, 2010 9:32 PM; 101 *days since my diagnosis.*

Hello everyone. This chemotherapy treatment was much better than the first, partly because I was more prepared, but also because it was just better. Not getting the shot the day after definitely helped.

First of all, I've realized I should not journal under the influence of chemotherapy. I really don't know what I'm saying, nor am I thinking straight. I didn't mean to share all the pain and side effects that I experienced the first time with chemo because I don't want people to worry. I shared more than I wanted to about my experience. With that being said, I tolerated the chemotherapy much better this time around. The bone pain was not as intense. There was/is still pain, but it is much, much more manageable. I can take an Advil and feel better after a little while.

The first week after chemotherapy drains me. Fatigue just takes over my body and there's not much I can do about it. On the second and third day, I can barely do anything. Somehow, I still manage to answer the phone and even have conversations with people. But by the next hour/day, I forget that I even talked to folk. I have to go through the call log on my phone to find out who I talked to or who texted me. However, with each day I am getting stronger. I am learning not to push myself too much and to pay attention to my body.

On chemotherapy day, I had the nerve to go to choir rehearsal. In my mind, I felt fine. But my memory...geesh. It takes a day before the drugs take effect. However, now I know next time I should not do that again. The drugs have me messed up.

Oh, before I forget, my medication was tweaked to prevent me from being nauseous. This drug is the same drug that gives me short-term memory loss. Instead of taking it for the three days, I only had to take it for one and one-half days unless I began to feel nauseous. This helped me be more present and aware as to what was going.

I am getting closer to the end of this cancer battle with each day passing. A few more months and I'll be done. During this time, me and my couch have really gotten to know each other pretty well. I'm sick of it and I'm sure it's sick of me. But we still have some more time together. I sit and binge watch television series all day and night. That's pretty much all I can do. However, if I'm having a good moment, I take full advantage of it and try to complete the things that I need to take care of (i.e. phone calls, etc.).

Before I go, I just wanted to share that one of my supporters has shaved off her hair, too. I told her in an earlier blog that it wasn't necessary, but she must've missed that post. Anyway, I appreciate your support (you know who you are), but please grow your hair....I'm trying to. It's cold outside. Speaking of which, my hair is growing back. There are a few strands coming in, and yes they're gray. My hair will probably fall out again next week, but at least I have some for now.

When we shaved off my hair a couple of weeks ago, it was liberating, but that feeling is so gone and I want some hair...now. I have yet to wear a wig. I tend to like the scarves better since I'm not used to having a lot of hair on my head.

To my shaved-head supporter and the rest of you, I appreciate you. This journey is still scary and I try to stay positive, but I still have my moments. Yet, through all of this, I am encouraged and strengthened from the love shown, your calls, texts, messages, etc. I just want to let you all know that I read everything that you write and I look forward to your encouraging words.

I just want to leave you all with a poem that was written for me by my friend, Michelle.

Just for You!

Can't ever begin to imagine
What you're going through
But our God he knows
And identifies with you.
He knows the pain
The doubt and the fear
He knows where you are
And bottles up each tear.
Put your head on his lap
Lay in his arms
Let Him hold you close
And rock you through the harm.
He's your Father, your friend
He's your husband ever true
All that He suffered,
He did it just for you.

Just for this moment
Especially for this time
Jesus loves you so much
He says I'm yours; you're mine.
Just for you; let Him hold your hand
Just for you Now
As you walk through this challenge
Let Him show you How.
Just for you!

Thank you, Michelle, for thinking about me and sending these words, just for me!

THURSDAY, JANUARY 21, 2010 11:26 PM; 105 *days since diagnosis.*

Time surely flies. I hadn't realized it's been since Sunday that I last wrote you all. There hasn't been a whole lot going on. I'm just trying to get my energy back. I had to go to the doctor's office (oncologist) on Tuesday because I have been having some issues with one of my fingers. After the first treatment, the skin on one of my fingertips began to peel. After a few days, it seemed to heal itself. However, after the second treatment, the same fingertip turned a purple-reddish color. Then the skin became hard around it and turned blue/green. It was crazy.

I figured I should let the doctor know about it since it wasn't a side effect listed on my sheet. They asked me to come into the office so that they could see exactly what I was talking about. It worked out great because I needed to have my blood drawn as well.

When I arrived at the office, there was a lady who was picking up a prescription of Oxycontin because of the excruciating bone pain that she was experiencing. I definitely could relate to her pain. I was just thankful I hadn't had bone pain like that since I refused the shot.

The nurse took my vitals and everything was okay. My temperature was a little elevated and so was my blood pressure, but nothing alarming. I let the nurse know I'd had my blood drawn earlier at the lab so that she look at the results and can see my blood count levels since I didn't get the shot. She looked at my numbers and told me my white blood cell count was really low. The nurse wasn't sure if I would have to get the shot or not. As you can imagine, I was not a happy camper.

When the doctor arrived, I figured I'd bring up other issues I was having with my treatment. Mind you, some side effects I was aware would occur, but some just didn't make sense to me or the doctor. I can't remember if I mentioned after my first treatment, I had a burn on my back. When I told the doctor, he didn't think it had anything to do with the chemotherapy drugs, but he couldn't explain it either. He thought maybe I had burned myself and I just forgot (because of the memory loss from the drugs). He never came right out and said that, but he didn't believe the burn came from chemotherapy. By the time I was able to show him the burn the first time, it had healed itself. This time, I had two burns on my back. The same location on either side. It was weird. Very weird. Since the blisters were still on my back this time, I was able to show the doctor and nurse, just in case they may've thought I was making this up, too...or at least overreacting. Still, the doctor doesn't understand why this is happening. He wants to keep an eye on them. At least he recognizes now that it's a side effect of the chemotherapy and not something I've done to myself. Hopefully, he'll be able to tweak some medications the next time.

There I was, two burns that couldn't be explained, a fingertip that couldn't be explained, and low white blood cells. I asked myself, "What is all of this?" A mess.

Fortunately, the doctor decided not to give me the

shot. He believes that my white blood cells level will rebound. If it doesn't by the time I go back for my next treatment, I may have to get the shot then. Right now, I have to keep a watch out for a fever. If my temperature goes above 100.5 degrees, I will have to let them know immediately and I may have to be monitored in the hospital. Needless to say, I am spending all of my time at home, away from crowds and away from germs.

I am so ready to be done with this. These past few months have been overwhelming. I know I'm halfway there, but the end still seems far away. Part of my concern is that my situation is taking its toll on one of my goddaughters/Raggedies, Aaliyah.

Last week, she brought home one of her school assignments where she had to write a story about what she did during her winter break. She talked about going sledding for the first time, taking family pictures, and giving presents to her family.

She also mentioned she went to spa for the first time and had her nails done. Then she wrote, "I went over my Auntie Andrea. She got cancer (two months ago). I feel bad for her." I wanted to cry knowing that she's even thinking about my situation at school. Every time I see or talk to her, she asks if the cancer is gone. Tonight, she said she wasn't even going to ask me what she wants to ask me because she already knows the answer. I told her, if she wants to ask, she can.

"Is it gone?"

I told her no, but that it was going away a little every day. Once before, I told her it'll be gone by her birthday, March 17th. I may've be a little presumptuous. But it would be great if it were. She said that would be the best birthday present ever. She told me she really wants it gone by February 30th. I let her know there were only twenty-eight days in February this year and there's never a 30th. She changed the subject (kind of) and asked me if I ate healthy fruits would the cancer go away then?

At the end of our conversation, she said, "I love you, Auntie Andrea." Usually, she would say, "I love you and I like you." Not this time. It's like she really wants me to know that she really loves me.

Anyway, I'm getting tired. I had a good evening watching the Cavaliers beat the Lakers (sorry Lakers fans). I will continue to pray for you all. Good night and God bless.

TUESDAY, JANUARY 26, 2010 9:24 PM; 110 days
since my diagnosis.

So here I am, just passing the days until my next
treatment, and what do I get in the mail? A bill. Not
just any bill, but my water bill. When I opened the
mail and saw how much I owed, my first thought
was, This can't be right. I need to call the water
department and let them know they made a mistake. Then I remembered "that" day. For those of you
who may not remember what happened "that" day,
it was the time when my mind was preoccupied and I
accidentally left my bathtub water running for hours
(I blogged about this before). I totally forgot about it
until today when I opened my bill. I used more water
in the months of October, November, and December than I did the entire spring and summer com-
bined...and that's with my sprinkler system running
twice a day. Oh well, what can I say? I have to be
thankful my ceiling didn't collapse or no other water
damage occurred.

Before I go, I'd like to share with you some quotes
that have been resonating with me. Enjoy...

"Life is not a matter of milestones, but of moments."
— Rose Kennedy

"Laugh as much as you breathe and love as long as you live." – Andrea Levy or Sherrilyn Kenyon or Johnny Depp or all of them

"Life is not about waiting for the storms to pass, it's about learning to dance in the rain." – Vivian Greene

Until next time, be blessed...

SUNDAY, JANUARY 31, 2010 10:52 PM; 115 *days since my diagnosis.*

Well, tomorrow is the day. I will have completed three of the four treatments. I'm excited knowing my chemo treatments are coming to an end in three more weeks.

––––––––

[personal reflection]

Yay. I was one step closer to being completely finished with chemo. I just wished the time would pass quicker. I was having unexplained side effects and one of my goddaughters was having a difficult time dealing with my cancer. It was easy to feel discouraged during this time. During this storm, I needed to figure out a way to dance in the rain. I needed encouragement.

I was blessed to have people who gave me encouraging words to ponder on. I was also thankful for the Word of God because it always gave me hope and encouraged my spirit. I had to appreciate and respect the process I was going through and make sure I made the most of each moment. I needed to laugh more and love more.

―――――――――

Reflection Questions

1. *How do you encourage yourself?*
2. *While going through a storm, how can you learn to dance in the rain?*
3. *How can you make each moment matter?*
4. *How can you learn to laugh and love more?*

12

chemo: round three

"IT IS A ROUGH ROAD THAT LEADS TO THE HEIGHTS
OF GREATNESS."

— LUCIUS ANNAEUS SENECA

———————

FRIDAY, FEBRUARY 5, 2010 12:05 PM; 120 days
since my diagnosis.

Whoa. This has been a rough week. I just wanted
to let you all know that I'm doing okay and hopefully
I'll have more energy next week to share my experience with my third chemo treatment. Love ya.

MONDAY, FEBRUARY 8, 2010 1:02 PM; 123 *days since my diagnosis.*

Hello everyone. I know it's been a while since I've been able to share, but as most of you suspected, this last chemo treatment kicked my butt. I couldn't get enough strength to even write. The treatments are definitely getting worse each time. Fortunately, I only have one more to go before surgery. I notice I tend to have more (and different) side effects with each session.

This time, I finally experienced the nausea I had previously escaped, and it was not good. But now, I'm back. Well, at least a little. My mind is much stronger, my body is stronger, but yet I still am fatigued. I can't even trick my body into believing that I have strength to do much. I get a good thirty minutes of energy before my body lets me know it's time to rest again. I am definitely getting my rest since I don't have a choice, and I'm drinking plenty of water to get these chemotherapy agents out of my system.

I want to share with you some things that happened last Sunday. First of all, one of my friends came by to visit with her boyfriend. I don't allow many visitors to come by because I don't want people sharing their germs and getting me sick...

Okay, I am going to have to continue this story later. I just received a call and I have to go to my doctor's office. They are concerned about the big bruise on my arm and they want me to come in to see what's going on. I'll be in touch later.

MONDAY, FEBRUARY 8, 2010 10:42 PM; 123 days since my diagnosis.

I'MMMMM BACKKKKKK! Okay, I guess I'll start with my visit today to the doctor's office. I had called my doctor earlier because I have a bruise on my arm where my IV was inserted last Monday. This was the first time that my body had reacted this way to the IV, and the area was dark red and very painful. I called the office to let them know and they wanted me to come in so they could make sure I didn't have an infection. Fortunately, I don't have an infection, but my doctor did say the area will get worse before it gets better. He said the bruised area will probably get bigger and then peel at some point. Thank God I only have one more treatment to go. I couldn't imagine having to do any more than that.

Unfortunately, I'm known as the problem child

at the doctor's office. Any time they talk about me they say, "If there's a side effect, Andrea will get it...and more." It's definitely the truth. Fortunately, the staff is awesome and they really take good care of me.

Besides the bruise, I was concerned about my fatigue. It's not just the normal fatigue. It's not like I can go to bed, rest, and then wake up feeling rejuvenated. When I go to sleep, I wake up still feeling fatigued. My doctor say it's part of the chemo process and I will have to deal with it until I'm finished and recovered.

My other issue is I feel like the chemo burned a hole in my stomach. This is new. Starting today, the doctor wants me to take some medication to help my stomach feel better, and he wants me to continue it until this side effect is gone. Also, I feel as though I can taste the chemo drugs, and not just the metallic taste, but worse. Gross.

My social worker overheard the conversation about my fatigue and gave me some information she thought would help. I told her I really want to be able to overcome the fatigue, but my body just says no. She suggested I meet with a physical therapist who specializes in helping cancer patients overcome the fatigue...well, at least empower them to overcome. I'm not exactly sure what the therapist would recommend, but I read exercise is supposed to help with fatigue. I'm not sure how it is supposed to work because when I climb a flight of stairs, I'm done. Totally exhausted. I tried to ride my stationary bike just to see if it helps, and I tell you, I felt more exhausted. Although, there are clinical studies that prove that exercise helps with the fatigue, I have to get enough energy before I can try to do at least 20 minutes.

While talking to the social worker about some of the other issues I experienced, she mentioned that I probably suffer from "chemo brain." Hearing her say that made me feel good, as crazy as that may sound. It lets me know my forgetfulness isn't all in my head. Chemo brain can be described as a mental cloudiness or fog caused by chemotherapy. I have been having issues remembering things and it's been very frustrating. I was forgetting things that happened yesterday and the day before. I have to write down everything that's important just in case I forget. Let me clarify. It's not that I forget everything, just some of the small details, but it's still aggravating. The doctor and social worker said that my memory will improve once chemo is over. Two weeks and then it's my final treatment.

I think I'll end my journal here for tonight, and tomorrow I'll finish my other story from earlier today. Sorry, I just can't write anymore.

TUESDAY, FEBRUARY 9, 2010 10:05 PM; 124 days since my diagnosis.

Well, just dropping in to say hi. I know I still need to complete my story from yesterday and share my experiences from my last chemo session, but today isn't the day. I will try again tomorrow. I am still dealing with my bruise which I now know is a burn, a "chemo burn."

A chemo burn occurs when some of the chemo agents escape into the skin at the IV injection site. I guess during the last chemo treatment, there must have been an issue with the placement of the IV and they didn't realize it. During the very first chemo treatment, there was a moment when I could feel the chemo burning as it was being administered and they adjusted the drip to slow down the process. I didn't have an issue during that time, well at least not at the injection site. You may recall I had burns on my back during the first two sessions. This time,

I had thought I'd escaped the burns because I didn't have any on my back, but now it's just my forearm. I guess this is just another issue that can happen with this process. Just when I thought it couldn't get any worse, it does. Anyway, I'm hoping this heals pretty well (and fast).

Even though I'm almost done with the chemo, the battle is not over. The end of this will be just the start of the next process. I still have to have surgery to remove the cancer. In case you forgot why I did chemo since I still have to have surgery to remove the tumor, the purpose is two-fold. First of all, the chemo is treating my entire body (systemically) in case there are any cancer cells that may have been somewhere else besides the breast. Secondly, the chemo is shrinking the cancer tumor. Therefore, depending on which surgery I have, they may only have to take out a small portion on my breast.

I shared with you before that the size of the cancer was a little over an inch. It's not considered large, but it's not small either. It would be great if the chemo was to shrink the cancer down to nothing, but from what I can tell, there is still a tumor there. I will go for testing next week to see exactly how much the tumor has been reduced. In the meantime, I have to get as

much information about the various surgery procedures that are available, because I have to decide
what I want to do next. I don't want to be deformed
after the surgery so I may have to do some reconstruction surgery. I don't know yet. Hopefully, things will
be as minimal as possible, but if you see me in some
DDs, then you'll know my decision.

There are a variety of factors that will come into
play in making my decision. However, the one thing
that is certain is that surgery will have to happen.
Hence, I am meeting with the plastic surgeon just in
case he is needed in this process.

All I can say is "Soon...."

FRIDAY, FEBRUARY 12, 2010 9:08 AM; 127 days
since my diagnosis.

Well my appointment with the plastic surgeon
yesterday was a bit premature again. The best time
for me to meet with him would be after my appointment with the surgeon. There are still so many
unknowns such as the size of the tumor, whether I
need radiation, the location of what's left of the
tumor, etc. However, it wasn't a total waste of time;
the plastic surgeon and I went over different scenar-
ios in order to give me an idea of what could be

involved in the reconstruction. If you recall from my last appointment with him, he had told me I had enough belly fat to do the one procedure where they take your stomach fat and vessels and put it in your breast. Well, I have good news (at least to me). When he grabbed my stomach fat, he told me I didn't have enough anymore. I tell you, there's nothing like having a guy grabbing at your belly fat. Meanwhile, just call me "Slim." LOL. However, he did say I have time and that he could fatten me up before the surgery. What? Is he serious? Who wants to get fattened up? I felt like a farm animal when he said that.

To make the most of my visit, I took the "Before" pictures...just in case. I can't wait to meet with the surgeon so that I can get a better understanding of my next steps and how much longer I'll be going through all of this. After that, I can finally make some decisions. I will keep you posted.

Andrea a.k.a. Slim

SUNDAY, FEBRUARY 21, 2010 12:26 PM; 136 days since my diagnosis.

I have not been in the mood to journal much since my last chemo treatment. I'm not sure if it's the chemo, but that's what I'm going to blame it on.

Anyway, tomorrow is my last day of chemo. I finally see a little light at the end of the tunnel. Of course, I am very excited, but as you can probably guess, I'm a little nervous, too. I know I've done this a few times already, but each time is different with different side effects. I don't know what to expect. Nonetheless, I think I'm going to go back to wearing my purple sweat suit for tomorrow. I may as well end treatments the same way as I began.

After tomorrow, I'll have more things to share with you.

I still haven't finished sharing my experiences and story from before. This is the continuation from my first blog on February 8th. It may seem like old news now, but I want to share. I will start the story again...just like I started it before:

Since my last "real" journal, a lot of things have crossed my mind that I wanted to journal about. At this point, I don't even remember everything, but there were a few things that happened last Sunday before my treatment that I wanted to share.

First of all, one of my friends and her boyfriend came by to visit. You already know, I don't really allow many visitors. Like I've said before, if I get a fever, I could spend days in the hospital. Anyway, I'll keep the names of my visitors anonymous since I'm sharing personal details, but it was a very nice visit. One of the purposes of the visit was for my friend to show her boyfriend my condominium community. He wanted to see my single-standing, detached condo. Once they arrived, we talked and I filled them in on my current breast cancer situation. My friend's boyfriend, newly named Chuck (I don't want to have to keep saying "my friend's boyfriend") shared with me that he is a breast cancer survivor.

––––––––––

[a quick reflection]

Prior to Chuck, I didn't know of any man who had been diagnosed with breast cancer besides Richard Roundtree, also known as Shaft. It was nice having Chuck over to talk about his journey because he has been where I am, even though he's a male. He was such a blessing and I appreciated him sharing his story. This is one of the reasons I don't mind sharing my story with people because I know I can be a blessing to someone else, too.

As an FYI, I want to share the following information about men and breast cancer. The American Cancer Society estimates breast cancer in men in the United States for 2015 are as follows:

- About 2,350 new cases of invasive breast cancer will be diagnosed.
- About 440 men will die from breast cancer.
- Breast cancer is about 100 times less common among men than among women.
- For men, the lifetime risk of getting breast cancer is about 1 in 1,000.
- The number of breast cancer cases in men relative to the population has been fairly stable over the last thirty years.

Men need to know that breast cancer is not limited to women. Possible symptoms of breast cancer to watch for include:

- A lump or swelling, which is usually (but not always) painless
- Skin dimpling or puckering
- Nipple retraction (turning inward)
- Redness or scaling of the nipple or breast skin
- Discharge from the nipple

Sometimes breast cancer can spread to lymph nodes under the arm or around the collar bone and cause a lump or swelling, even before the tumor is large enough to be felt. These changes aren't always caused by cancer. Still, if you notice any breast changes, you should see your health care professional as soon as possible. Okay, now back to the blog...

CON'T OF SUNDAY, FEBRUARY 21, 2010 BLOG...

Chuck's experience with chemotherapy and surgery were very similar to mine. He had his tumor surgically removed after his chemo treatment. Since it's rare for men to get breast cancer, the physicians didn't really know how to treat Chuck post-chemo and post-surgery. They didn't know whether to give him hormone therapy or not since he was a male. I can't remember if he had to take them or not. Fortunately, he is healthy once again.

Before Chuck left, he asked if he could pray with/ for me. I thought to myself, "How sweet."

I said, "Of course you can."

He told me he prays for me every morning. How sweet it that, too? You never know who is lifting you up in prayer. This is how we should be as Christians. It is our responsibility to help those who need help. To pray for those who need our prayers.

During his prayer, he asked God to give me the desires of my heart. Hearing that really pulled on my heart strings because my favorite Bible verse is Psalms 37:4 (NIV), "Delight thyself also in the Lord and he shall give thee the desires of thine heart." The following verse says, "Commit thy way unto the Lord: trust also in him; and he shall bring it to pass." What a powerful Word from God and how appropriate during this time.

I feel it was important to share this story about Chuck so you are aware that breast cancer is not just a woman's issue. Men can get it, too.

After my girlfriend and Chuck left, I received another visit from Leighton (a.k.a. Neighbor) and his 1-year old daughter. His daughter, who I call Sunshine, recently had open-heart surgery to correct some defects. Even though she and I were both dealing with major health issues, it was very difficult processing that this little baby had to have major surgery. Being so young, she didn't understand what was going on and how serious her situation was. I'm tearing up just thinking about the conversation I had with Neighbor when I found out. My heart was broken when I heard the news. It was a difficult time, especially for her parents. I tried to be strong for my friends even though I was a mess on the inside.

Through prayers and the grace of God, Sunshine came out of her surgery much better than expected.

Although Leighton brought Sunshine over to visit me, she was more intrigued with my dog, Gigi. Sunshine had never been around a dog and was fascinated with this new "thing." Gigi is a Yorkshire Terrier who weighs about seven and one-half pounds. She's a dog who believes she's a baby, too.

Sunshine kept chasing her, trying to pick her up, but Gigi was too excited and kept running around the house. She jumped from my lap to Neighbor's lap and then all around the floor. When Sunshine saw Gigi running around everywhere, she became tickled. She kept laughing. Her laugh was so cute and infectious. It was a pleasure to watch her fascinated with Gigi. It was precious. In that moment, I realized how important it is to enjoy life, enjoy the moments. "Life is not a matter of milestones, but of moments."

I call Leighton's daughter Sunshine because she brightens my day. With everything she's been through in her short life, it's great to see her appreciate the simple things in life and find joy in watching a dog run around the house. She let Gigi lick her hands. She pulled on Gigi's ear. She had a good time. In all of this, Sunshine reminded me that I, too, will be appre-

ciative of the simple things and find joy again. By the
way, I was so proud of my Gigi for being such a "good
girl" in all of this. She hasn't been around too many
babies before and I wasn't sure how she would act.

I hope this blog was an easy read. I don't have
the energy to read it and make sure it flows correctly.
However, before I leave, I'll just give you a quick
update on my last appointment with the surgeon.

Last Tuesday, I met with my surgeon. Before the
appointment, I had to have another mammogram
and ultrasound of my right breast. They wanted to
compare the results to the previous one. It was difficult for me to see anything on the mammogram, I
didn't see much shrinkage of the tumor. I was a little bummed, but when I met with the doctor, she said
that the tumor did shrink. That made me feel better. We talked about my options again: a lumpectomy with six weeks of radiation, five times a week,
about ten minutes each day OR a mastectomy (without radiation).

Regardless, my blood levels need to get better
before I can have surgery, so it will probably not happen until late March, early April. I still have some
time to decide what my next steps are going to be. I've
been procrastinating on this decision. I am just pray-

ing for clarity so I can make the right decision for me. We'll see what happens. Anyway, I am reaching the point of delirium, so I'm going to say good night and I'll talk to you tomorrow hopefully.

———

[personal reflection]

Finally, the light at the end of the tunnel. There was only one more chemo treatment. The road hadn't been easy but I welcomed the challenged and fought this thing that was trying to destroy me head-on.

At times, I felt like I was in school again. There was so much I didn't know and I had to continuously learn about this disease and the various treatment plans. I had to be educated in order to be victorious.

Also, as mentioned in the blog, I hadn't personally known any man who had gone through breast cancer prior to Chuck. I shared his story to reinforce the fact that breast cancer is not just a women's disease. It's a human disease. Men, check your man boobs, too, even if you don't have much breast tissue.

———

Reflection Questions

1. *What or who is your "Sunshine" that brightens your day?*

2. *When faced with a difficult situation, how do you persevere?*

3. *To both women and men, have you performed your monthly breast exam?*

13

chemo: round four

"THERE WILL COME A TIME WHEN YOU BELIEVE
EVERYTHING IS FINISHED. YET THAT WILL BE THE
BEGINNING."

— LOUIS L'AMOUR

TUESDAY, FEBRUARY 23, 2010 10:38 PM; 138
days since my diagnosis.

I finally have enough energy to share my experience with my final chemo treatment yesterday. I was
excited when I arrived at the clinic for my last chemo

session ever. This was it! After all of the months, I will be done with chemotherapy. I will have to see my oncologist on a regular basis, but I don't have to sit in my chemo treatment room anymore.

The process started out normal. I received the steroid, anti-nausea medication, and Pepcid through the IV. Once this was done, it was now time for the chemo agents. Both agents were supposed to take about 1 hour each to be administered. As the first drug was dripping into my veins, I noticed a new side effect I hadn't noticed before, I was having chest and abdominal pains. *Shaking My Head* I called for the nurse and after she spoke to the doctors, they decided to stop the IV until the symptoms left.

Next, my acid reflux began to bother me. If you've never experienced acid reflux, be glad. Acid reflux can occur when the valve between the esophagus and stomach doesn't close all the way and the acid in the stomach move back up into the esophagus. Reflux can cause burning chest pain (a.k.a. heartburn). I had to take some Maalox to get it together.

After all of that, I began to cough uncontrollably. The doctor would not start chemo until I stopped coughing, so I had to suck on a Hall's cough drop in order to control it. Instead of IV dripping for the hour, they slowed down the rate to two hours. It seemed to take forever, but fortunately, I didn't have any other complications from that agent.

For the next chemo agent, the process went off without a hitch and only took an hour. By the time I was finished with this session, I had been there for a total of six hours. I guess this last treatment wanted to make itself memorable.

Before I left, the nurse gave me a brochure on how to cope after chemotherapy and a pin that said, "Never place a period where God has placed a comma!" I appreciated those words of encouragement. It's a reminder that it's not over until God says it's over.

Today, I feel just okay. I don't have much energy and I'm back to only eating crackers and drinking ginger ale. It feels great knowing I don't have to do another treatment. Now, I am waiting until I begin to feel better and get stronger. From past experience, I know these first few days are challenging, but I will hopefully start getting better by Saturday.

MONDAY, MARCH 8, 2010 9:32 PM; 151 days since my diagnosis.

Hey there. It's been almost two weeks since I last blogged. I needed a break. Just like before, I had a pretty rough time after the last chemo treatment. I am feeling much better now. This was the first time I didn't call the doctor's office about my side effects. However, I have been having some weird side effects. My right eye and both legs have been twitching for a few days. Also, my stomach feels like it's twitching, too. I'm hoping this will pass soon. If it's not gone by my next appointment, I'll bring it up at that point. I am happy I don't have to do this chemo anymore. It is over. Now, I'm waiting for surgery. I know you all are probably wondering what surgery I'm going to have, but I'll get to that later.

First, I want to take you back a couple of weeks. The Saturday following my last chemo treatment, Nakia gave her dog, Cola, a birthday party. Cola had turned 1 year old and to celebrate, she was having a party/play date with Gigi. Nakia came over and picked up Gigi and they "partied" and had pupcakes. When she dropped Gigi off, Nakia looked at me and said, "Are you losing your eyebrows?" I told her I wasn't, but that I had shaped them earlier. However, after she left, I looked in the mirror again and realized my brows did look sparser.

"Oh no, I am losing my eyebrows."

Throughout this process, I was happy I hadn't lost my eyebrows or eyelashes. I felt that losing either would make me look sick. However, now, after my last treatment, my eyebrows and eyelashes were disappearing. The good thing is they should grow back soon...at least I hope. I find myself being more cautious as I wash my face because every strand counts. I am so ready for my hair to grow back so I can look like my old self. Things should be back to normal by the summer.

Before I make my final decision about my surgery, I want to make sure I am fully informed about the risks and benefits of each of my options. Last week, I met with a radiation oncologist to learn more about radiation therapy. I've read/heard so many different stories about radiation that I just felt it would be better if I would get the information for myself. My biggest fear was being burned, but I found out that there were other potential side effects that were concerning to me; I could experience fatigue, loss of appetite, thickening of the skin, discoloration, and possibly fluid build-up.

I've discussed with you before that I can either choose to do a lumpectomy with radiation or have a mastectomy, which won't require radiation. Regardless, there is no difference in survival between the two choices. The decision is up to me. It's really what I'm most comfortable with. I'm giving myself until Friday to decide which surgery I'm going to do. Either way, my surgery will be some time in the beginning of April. The doctor wants to wait until my body is healthy again.

Right now, I'm trying to fight this fatigue so I can get back to some normalcy. I have a few more appointments before surgery. I have to meet with my oncologist and eye doctor again next week. The floater in my eye seems to be gone, but it's hard to tell for sure. If not, it's definitely much smaller.

I know I sound like a broken record because I say this all the time, but I want you all to know that I really feel all of your prayers. Take care and love y'all.

SATURDAY, MARCH 20, 2010 9:30 AM; 163 *days since my diagnosis.*

Time is just passing by. I didn't realize that it's been almost two weeks since I last wrote on my blog. Since the last time, there has been some new information. My surgery is finally scheduled for April 12th.

I know you are probably wondering which surgery, lumpectomy or mastectomy, but believe it or not, I have not made up my mind 100 percent. I was supposed to decide last Friday. Then I gave myself the deadline of yesterday. I just need to write down the pros and cons, risks and benefits, and then determine what I'm going to do. But at least I have a date scheduled. I should be back to my "new" normal in no time...at least by May.

Since my last blog, I had an appointment with my oncologist. He said I'm doing fine. My chemo burns have healed. Now, I just have the scars as a reminder. My biggest concern that I brought to his attention was my fatigue. It's amazing how I can get tired at a drop of a dime. I really can't wait to feel like I use to, but I realize it's going to take some time. My other side effect concerns were answered with "they'll get better in time." Because the effects of chemo are cumulative, it is common to be more fatigued or continue to experience side effects after completing the treatments. I've been drinking plenty of water to try to get these chemo agents out of my system.

I found out that for the next couple of years, I will have to meet with my oncologist every three months. My next appointment with him is two weeks after my surgery. The purpose of the visit is so I can get my prescription for Tamoxifen. Tamoxifen is a chemo drug which interferes with the activity of estrogen. The type of cancer I have thrives on estrogen, so the goal of the Tamoxifen is to be an antagonist and prevent the cancer from coming back. I will have to take this drug for the next five years. I just pray I don't experience any negative side effects from it. My doctor wants me to start the drug the week after surgery, but I don't even know how I'll be feeling at that time. I asked if I could wait a little longer, so he gave me the additional week. Honestly, I wasn't quite ready to hear about the Tamoxifen because I still haven't decided about my surgery. One step at a time. I've been trying to take this journey in stages. It keeps me from being overwhelmed and stressed.

Yesterday, I had a follow-up appointment with my eye doctor. My doctor said my eyes looked "gorgeous" and everything was fine. I have to go back in a few months just to make sure nothing changes. I was glad to hear that. I was going to entertain you all and journal with my eyes dilated again. However, because the wait time for my appointment was so long, by the time I was in front of my computer again, I could see the keyboard just fine.

With everything that has been going on, some-how I forgot that I have a friend who is a plastic surgeon. I reached out to him to get his perspective about my surgery. Unbeknownst to me, he specializes in breast reconstruction. He has been a great resource in helping me make my decision about surgery by giving his perspective about the benefits and risks.

I am still singing in the church choir. We are learning a new song, "Everything is Changed," by Youthful Praise. Every time I hear that song, it just makes me think about my life and how everything has changed. Five months ago, I would've never thought I would be in a battle for my life right now. Everything has changed. The person I was before that October 8th, I will never be again.

Fortunately, I'm finally getting closer to the end of this battle. Praise God. I realize this cancer "experience" didn't just happen to me. It happened to everyone who cares about me. I want to thank you all for riding this journey with me. I don't know exactly where it'll lead me/us, but I know good things are to come. So once again, thanks. I love you all for being there for me.

Andrea a.k.a Ann a.k.a Dre', a.k.a Mook a.k.a Dyan a.k.a Drea a.k.a. Slim

THURSDAY, APRIL 1, 2010 9:25 AM; 175 *days since my diagnosis.*

We are now in the month of April...11 more days until my surgery. No, I haven't made a decision about my reconstruction yet. It's coming soon.

Happy Birthday, Jackie...40 years old today.

MONDAY, APRIL 12, 2010 12:45 AM; 186 *days since my diagnosis; approximately 12 hours before surgery*

I'm trying not to cry too much but as I write this I can't help it. I'm crying because I can't believe the day is finally here. Hopefully and prayerfully this is my last day with cancer forever. This whole process has been a roller coaster. Ups and downs, back and forth. The only thing that hasn't changed is God's grace and mercy. I can't wait until the next time I can write you all. I will be cancer-free!

My surgery is scheduled for today at 12:30 p.m. I had to stop my eating at midnight and I hope I don't get too hungry while I'm waiting. When I'm hungry is when I get irritable. As I wrote that, I had to laugh out loud because that's the least of my worries. I will have to stay in the hospital overnight, but other than that, I'm not sure about the next steps. I know I will have drains this time, so it'll take some time for recuperation.

I don't have a song on the top of my head or in my heart right now, but I do want to go back to my favorite saying, "Through all of this mess, there's a gift to be found." There've been many gifts throughout all of this. I've learned so much about myself through this process, even though I thought I knew myself pretty well after thirty-nine years. God is something else. It's amazing how He uses all of our circumstances for good. As I mentioned before (I think), I've never asked the question "why me?" nor will I. It really doesn't matter at this point because it is me. I will admit I still can't believe this is my life. I just hope through all of this, I get out of this what I'm supposed to and that I don't lose it.

Well, that's it for now. I'm sleepy and getting a little nervous as I think about my surgery. I hope I can fall asleep.

WEDNESDAY, APRIL 14, 2010 8:21 PM; *188 days since my diagnosis.*

I came home today. Doing okay. I'll provide an update when I'm feeling a little better.

[personal reflection]

As I read this journal update on my blog, I remember how overly excited and grateful I was to be cancer-free. Surgery was over and now I could begin to find my "new" normal. Even though I may not have questioned why me, I still didn't understand why. Well, maybe I did understand. I needed to change. I needed to find my purpose.

I never doubted I would be able to handle whatever came my way but I would be telling a fib if I said this journey wasn't going to be challenging. It was. However, I built a lot of character going through this battle and I hope the person I became as a result of this journey stays with me forever.

Reflection Questions

1. *What challenging situation have you encountered that has helped you build character?*

2. *What are three character traits you want others to associate with you?*

14

I'm a conqueror!

IN ALL THESE THINGS WE ARE MORE THAN
CONQUERORS THROUGH HIM WHO LOVED US.

— ROMANS 8:37

TUESDAY, APRIL 20, 2010 4:41 PM; *194 days since
my diagnosis.*

*Today, I received the news that I've been waiting
to hear since October 8, 2009. I am CANCER-
FREE. Hearing this and saying it, is emotional for*

me. *I've been fighting this battle to the best of my ability, and now I have victory. Thank you, Jesus! It was a scary road to travel, but I didn't doubt the outcome during the journey. I am in awe of God's grace and how He's brought me through this. I don't have to do anymore chemotherapy nor any radiation. My margins were free and clear. This means the tissue surrounding the edge of the tumor didn't contain any cancer cells. Now, I have to meet with my oncologist so that I can start Tamoxifen for the next five years. As you may recall, Tamoxifen is a drug that is used to block the actions of estrogen and to prevent some types of breast cancer. I will get back to you all at a later time to let you know about how the surgery went and the recovery phase. I'm out of energy right now. Just know that your prayers worked.*

[a quick reflection]

Before I started fighting this battle, I must admit I was scared. Scared of the unknown. Scared of dying. I realize that it was natural to feel fear, but I couldn't live in it. I acknowledged it, prayed on it, prayed through it, and then put my trust in God. Sometimes, as I reflect on all that I've been though, I just shake my head. This has been a heck of a journey. But thanks be to God, I made it through. I am more than a conqueror.

I was blessed throughout my battle. Most people didn't even know I was fighting for my life. I remember leaving church one day and a member of the church complimented me on how my scarves always coordinate with my outfits. I just smiled. He didn't know the scarves weren't for fashion, but were a necessity to cover my bald head. I didn't look like someone who was going through cancer, well what most people perceive people with cancer to look like. Sometimes you can't tell who's fighting this battle. There were times where I went to my appointments and/or treatments and I would see someone who looked like they were battling cancer. All I could do is pray...and praise.

> *"Give thanks to the Lord, for he is good; his love endures forever." –* 1 Chronicles 16:34 *(NIV)*

I praise God because He continues to be faithful to me. I pray I never have to go to through it again. Although there were some hiccups along the way, I came out on top. I'm alive!

In my strong alto voice, I'm singin',

> *Praise God, from whom all blessings flow;*
> *Praise Him, all creatures here below;*

Praise Him above, ye heav'nly host;
Praise Father, Son, and Holy Ghost. [3]

This doxology, or short hymn, was written in 1674 by Thomas Ken. Three hundred and fifty years later, these words continue to move me. I will continue to praise God for who He is and what He's done in my life. He has allowed me to go through this journey and now, I can declare that I am cancer-free.

As the American Cancer Society would say, today is my birthday! This is the day to start with a new slate and truly start living my life. A life transformed by breast cancer.

Breast cancer is a yucky disease and unfortunately, there are too many people who are affected by it. According to research, one in eight women in the U.S. will be diagnosed with breast cancer in her lifetime. Let's just take that in for a moment. Say you're in a room with eighty women, ten of them will be diagnosed with breast cancer. If it's a room of twenty-four women, three of them will be diagnosed in their lifetime. Just take a moment and think of sixteen women who are close to you. According to the statistics, two of them will be diagnosed with breast cancer in their lifetime. This statistic is staggering to me. For women in the age range of 40-59, breast cancer is the leading cause of cancer death in the U.S. I was only 39 years old when I was diagnosed.

I knew of other women who battled breast cancer, but it was always those women over there. Those who were far removed from me. It wasn't something I ever thought could happen to me. My grandmother had been diagnosed eight years prior to me, but she was 85 years old. Her doctor mentioned that most older people will eventually end up with some form of cancer, so he didn't think it was genetic. Actually, only five to ten percent of breast cancers in the U.S. are due to inherited mutations in the BRCA1 or BRCA2 breast cancer genes. As you may recall, I was tested to see if I carried these two genes and the results came back negative. I mean, do we really know what causes breast cancer? Hopefully, we'll have an answer to that question during my lifetime.

Overall, breast cancer is second only to lung cancer in cancer deaths among women in the U.S. That is scary. Statistics show a woman is diagnosed with breast cancer every two minutes, and a woman dies of breast cancer every thirteen minutes. This is not just a woman's issue, though. As I mentioned earlier, men can be affected, too. Compared to an estimated 292,130 women diagnosed with breast cancer in 2015, there were 2,350 men diagnosed. An estimated 40,290 women and 440 men will die from breast cancer in the U.S. in 2015. The good thing, *if there is anything good about breast cancer,* is the five-year survival rate for breast cancer is 99 percent if it's caught early. That's why it's so important to get to know your breasts. Stay aware...

———————————

SUNDAY, APRIL 25, 2010 11:35 PM; 199 days since my diagnosis.

Hey y'all. I just wanted to touch base with you while I was having a good moment. My recovery from surgery is going slower than I would like. I have two drains that I can't wait to get removed. The drains are used to remove excess body fluid that accumulates at the surgical site. The fluid is collected in a soft, round squeeze bulb that looks like a grenade. Tomorrow, I'm going to call and see if I can get them out. I think/hope that I'll feel much better once the drains are gone. However, I need to have less than 30 cc of fluids collected for two days before the doctor will remove the drains. Thank goodness, I'm almost there.

I want to share with you what's been going on over the past couple of weeks. As you know, I had my surgery on April 12th. You may be wondering which surgery I had, lumpectomy versus mastectomy. It was definitely a tough decision to make, but I needed to choose the one that I could be at peace with.

I chose to have the mastectomy...a double mastectomy. I know some of you are wondering why I went to the extreme with my decision, but I can tell you, I don't want to ever hear that I have cancer again. Ever. I want to minimize the possibility of having breast cancer again, in either breast. Last week when I met with the surgeon, she asked how I felt about my decision. I don't have any regrets about my decision (even with the pain). Plus, there's no going back now. I know I made the best decision for me. Being able to talk with other women who have gone through this was helpful in making my decision.

After the surgery, I spent two nights in the hospital. I felt pretty good, considering. I had a lot of visitors which was nice. My second night at the hospital, people brought me some of my favorites: spinach dip (thanks, Neighbor), Synder's Bar-B-Q chips, and collard greens (thanks, Terri). After being able to eat all of that and not puking, I knew everything was uphill from that point.

Once I made it home, I spent a lot of time sleeping in my cozy chair in the living room. It was easier to sleep upright and not have to worry about accidentally rolling onto my surgical site or pulling out the drains.

My aunt Lois stayed with me until that Friday night because my mom was under the weather. It would've been pitiful with both of us not feeling well trying to take care of each other. My mom came over and stayed with me on Friday night and my grandmother joined us on Saturday.

It was nice having them around to help me as I recuperated. I thought it was cute that every night when my 93.5-year-old grandmother would go to bed, she would say, "I'm about to go to sleep now. Ain't you ready to go to sleep, too?" I would tell her, "No, I'm not, Woman," and then she would kiss my 'not-so-bald' head and say, "May God bless and keep you," and then go upstairs to bed.

My mom kept suggesting that I try sleeping in my bed. After a while, I decided to give it a try. About 7:00 a.m., I heard my grandmother coming into my room to check on me. She would come in and look at me, but never said a word. She was funny. But what's even funnier is when I started sleeping upstairs, she felt that when she went to bed, everybody should go to bed. Every night, I found myself chuckling when she would say it's time to go to bed. It wasn't worth me *trying to explain that I was grown and I wasn't ready to go to bed, so I got up and went to bed when she did.*

My mom shared with me that when she was a child and my grandmother was ready to go to sleep, she would turn the TV off, and tell everyone in the house that they had to go to sleep, too. You gotta love her. I must admit, it was great having time with both my mother and grandmother. Even though, I felt as though I could take care of myself, I really couldn't. I couldn't cook for myself or do anything more than sleep and rest.

Last Tuesday, I had my appointment with the breast surgeon. That's when I received the news that I was cancer-free. Yay! Thursday, I met with the plastic surgeon to see when I could start the next phase of reconstructive surgery. Nothing can get started until the drains are out and my scars are healed.

[personal reflection]

Surgery was over. It was both good and bad. Good that the cancer was gone. Bad because so were my boobs. Once my breasts were removed, I wasn't sure how I would feel. I didn't know if I would feel as though I suffered a loss or if I'd feel as though part of my femininity would be gone. Surprisingly, I was okay. I think I had prepared myself for this moment, plus the cancer was gone. Instead of focusing on the loss of my breasts, I choose to focus on what I gained...life.

God has shown me over and over again that He is truly faithful. I'm so grateful for the stronger, deeper relationship that I have with Him. I will never be the person that I was before cancer; I was transformed.

This new me is taking some getting used to. By no means am I complaining because I have so much to be thankful for. As a result of this journey, I emerged stronger, wiser, more faithful, more appreciative, more mature, more giving, more resilient, more beautiful – inside and out – and, just *more*.

I was not finished with the process; this was just the first phase of the reconstruction. During this time, I needed to continue to recuperate. I was ecstatic that I didn't have cancer inside of my body trying to destroy me. I was able to rest easier knowing that I was healthy once again.

Reflection Questions

1. *What obstacles have you overcome/conquered?*
2. *What "more" did you become during the process?*

3. *What did you have to risk to win?*

15

life after cancer

"LIFE IS A SONG — SING IT. LIFE IS A GAME — PLAY IT. LIFE IS A CHALLENGE — MEET IT. LIFE IS A DREAM — REALIZE IT. LIFE IS A SACRIFICE — OFFER IT. LIFE IS LOVE — ENJOY IT."

— SAI BABA

WEDNESDAY, MAY 5, 2010 11:27 AM; 209 days since my diagnosis.

"Nature does not hurry, yet everything is accomplished." – Lao Tzu.

That quote is so true. Those words were on the cover of a card I received from one of my co-workers. The timing was perfect because I was beginning to feel better and was trying to do more than I should. Maybe I'll try to drive. Maybe I'll get on my recumbent exercise bike. Or maybe I will vacuum my living room floor. Even though I felt better, I remembered what happened when I did too much, too soon after the lymph node surgery. During that time, I was calling/interrupting my doctor while she was on vacation because I thought I messed something up.

I opened to the inside of the card and it read, "Take time to nurture your soul and yourself." I have to keep in mind that I cannot rush my healing process. I have to take it in stride. Even though the healing process seems long and slow, I realize once it's done, I will be fully healed. If I try to do too much, too soon, it may prolong all of this. "Nature does not hurry, yet everything is accomplished." As you can see, I have to keep saying it to myself because it's hard for me to rest and be patient with my recovery.

Each day is better than the previous one. I have arm exercises that I have to do so I don't get a "frozen" arm. I haven't begun driving yet, but I'm hoping to test out my skills soon...maybe. I think the last time I blogged, I still had my drains. Those came out last week and I feel much better without them. Now, I'm just waiting for the incisions where the drains were to heal. I don't have much energy, but I try to walk to my mailbox each day.

In May, I'm supposed to walk in my first breast cancer walk as a survivor. My cousin, Terri put together Team Mook (my nickname from when I was a child) and a bunch of us will walk a mile on Mother's Day. I don't think a mile will be too much for me; I will walk it slowly. I hope the weather cooperates with us. Cleveland weather is so unpredictable that it very well may rain or even snow on that day.

I have a friend/co-worker who participated in the Avon 2-Day walk in Washington D.C. this past weekend. Her goal was to "beat cancer one step at a time." The walk was a total of 39.9 miles and she raised almost three thousand dollars for breast cancer research. I was so honored that she chose to walk in celebration of me. She and chose me as one of her "She-Roes."

Oh, I forgot to mention that last week, I started on my 5-year drug, Tamoxifen. So far, so good. I haven't had any side effects yet. I pray things will continue to go well. My doctor mentioned the main side effects are weight gain and hot flashes. However, I only have to take it for five years, and I already have one week down. Only two hundred and fifty-nine weeks to go.

Anyway, that's it for now. I had to share on my blog today because I received word that my aunt and her co-workers think I'm slacking with my postings and that I need to write more often. I know my blogs have become more infrequent, but it's only because I don't have much to say now. I sleep, eat, rest, sleep, eat, rest, watch TV, go to doctor's appointments, eat, sleep and repeat. I will keep you all updated with major things that come up. You all have been with me from the beginning of this, so you may as well stay with me 'til the end of the process. I'm hoping it won't be too long though. Tomorrow is my first "real" reconstruction appointment with my plastic surgeon.

FRIDAY, MAY 14, 2010 5:36 PM; *218 days since my diagnosis.*

Hello all. I hope each one of you had a good week. Mine has been okay. Physically, I'm getting stronger each day and I'm feeling pretty good about my memory/mind. I've been able to do some technical training for work and it went well. Unfortu-

nately, there has been one pressing issue. I have been having a really bad headache on the top of my head for the past three days. I don't know what caused this. It reminds me of the pain I felt when I had the bone pain during chemotherapy. I'm not sure if the pain is caused by the Tamoxifen, but my doctor told me to stop taking it for the next two weeks. We'll see what happens.

Since our last talk, I participated in my first breast cancer walk as a survivor. It was The Race at Legacy Village on Mother's Day. The mile-long run/walk was fun even though it was cold outside. I got my face painted with the breast cancer ribbon on both cheeks. The run started at 9:00 a.m. and my uncle and cousins ran the mile. After they were done, the walk started. All the walkers walked around Legacy Village together. It was a great time being there with loved ones. I still wasn't very strong physically, but walking the mile wasn't too bad. However, after I came home, I took a nap for two and one-half hours.

I want to send a big thank you to Terri for putting this together. For those of you who have fussed at me because I didn't tell you about the walk, I apologize. However, you will have the opportunity to walk in celebration with me at the Race for the Cure on September 11th. Currently, I'm trying to think of a team name for the walk. If anyone has any suggestions, please let me know. I will post the information on the site if you would like to join my team or make a donation to the cause. So far, I've had the following suggestions for the team name: The Awesomes (by my Raggedy, Aaliyah) and the A-Team.

Also, I have a sorority sister/friend who is participating in the American Cancer Society's Relay for Life in Dallas. She called and asked if I would mind if she wore a banner with my name on it. Of course I don't mind. She will be wearing a banner in honor of me being a survivor. I feel so special to have all these people thinking of me and walking in honor of me.

Okay, getting back to my physical condition. As I mentioned, I'm doing well for the most part. I went to the plastic surgeon's office for my first expansion. When I had the mastectomy, expanders were implanted so my muscle and skin could be stretched to form new boobs. The expanders are kind of like implants with a little saline. At each doctor's visit, the expander gets injected with more saline until the desired size is obtained.

You may wonder how this is done. The expander

has a magnet in it which helps locate the port where the saline is injected into the expanded. The doctor uses another magnet to find where the port is located and then saline is injected. The amount of saline varies depending on how much I can take. The surgeon doesn't want to give me too much saline; that could be unbearable.

After the injection, the expanders are a little painful. The pain only lasts for a couple of days. Right now, I'm going every two weeks for my injections, but I believe after my next one, they'll change my schedule so that I can do weekly injections.

Once the injections are completed, I'll have surgery to have the expanders removed and implants will be put in their place. I'm not sure how long this process is going to take. It can be anywhere from two months to...I don't know. I guess we'll have to see. As always, I'll keep you all posted.

Again, please keep in mind the Race for the Cure in September. I would love for you all to join me in the fight against breast cancer. Besides me, I'm sure many of you know others who have been touched by breast cancer.

My cousin, Adrienne mentioned she would like for my 93.7-year-old grandmother to come to the

Race for the Cure and participate this year. I think that's a great idea. Of course, my grandmother will not be participating as a walker, but she will represent as a survivor. We will have to figure out how to make this work.

Before I go, I wish all the mothers out there a belated Happy Mother's Day!

TUESDAY, JUNE 1, 2010 4:49 PM; *236 days since my diagnosis.*

I went back to work last week just to see how it would go. I did well, even though I ran out of steam earlier in the day than I would've liked. I have learned to be patient while I'm building up my stamina again. Working definitely exposed some residual issues I have from chemo. The main thing is my short-term memory. It sucks. I have to write things down just to make sure I don't forget them. I went to the doctor today and he told me it'll get better. I asked how long and he said, "Well studies show improvement after one year and back to normal after two years."

Seriously? One year shows improvement? Two years to get back to normal? That long, huh? The doctor said there's not any medicine that can help with the memory loss, but I am going to figure out something soon.

This past weekend, I went to visit my family in Roanoke, VA. I thought I was sneaking into town to surprise my dad, but someone had told him I was coming. It was all good though because I really wanted him to see I was doing fine now. I know he worries about me, especially since I'm so far away. It was a great visit. I was able to see mostly everyone I wanted. However, I was worn out hanging with all my family...especially the little ones.

While I was there, I found out that another family member is going through the same thing. She is currently done with her chemotherapy treatments now, but her surgery isn't until Thursday. She told me she uses my blog as inspiration. I'm glad to know that my blog is of good use and helping others.

The main reason I wanted to write this blog today was to inform you all about the team that I formed for the Race for the Cure. I plan on walking the 5K on September 11th. This 5K walk will be different for me because with each step toward the finish line, I will be walking toward my new role in life, finding a cure. I would love for each of you to cross the finish line with me. You all have been an instrumental part of this journey and this is a great way to finish it together. Also, this will be my first fundraiser attempt as a survivor. The cost to participate is twenty dollars and you will receive a T-shirt and a bib. We desperately have to find a cure and in order to do that, more research is needed. Chemo sucks! Mastectomy sucks! Radiation sucks! New, bigger boobs...well that might not be too bad. We'll see...LOL. But seriously, together, with your support, we can do our part in finding a cure.

TUESDAY, JULY 6, 2010 5:55 PM; 271 days since my diagnosis.

Hey Strangers. It's been a while since we last spoke. I hope you had a great Fourth of July. I really enjoyed my holiday weekend. Now, I'm just preparing to hang out with my family at our reunion next weekend. Also, I'll be celebrating my 40th birthday. I tell you, I'm so looking forward to this birthday. I'm so ready to put this past year behind. Needless to say, I had a lot going on in my thirty-ninth year. However, I am thankful to just be "living." Going through cancer is difficult because you never know which end of the spectrum you'll end up on. Life or death. I just thank God for life...even though it's forever different.

With that being said, I am planning a "Celebration of Life" party on Saturday, August 7th. The location will be at my home. I would love for you all to join me as I celebrate my life...all forty years of it. Please let me know if you think you can make it so I can have an accurate count for the number of guests.

P.S. Just in case you all are curious how things are going with me and my boobs, things are progressing. I still don't know when my reconstructive surgery will happen. Right now, I'm still in the process of getting expanded and yes, it hurts. As always, I'll keep you posted.

WEDNESDAY, AUGUST 11, 2010 4:57 PM; 307 days since my diagnosis.

Hey there, everyone. I hope this journal update finds you well. As for me, I'm doing great. I am still on cloud nine from my Celebration of Life party last Saturday. Since I wasn't sure how the weather was going to be, I rented a tent, table, and chairs and had them set up in the park area in front of my home. The tables were decorated with fuchsia tablecloths and balloons to match.

I decided to have the party catered so I wouldn't have to worry about preparing the food. The caterer and his staff were awesome. They cooked delicious food, served it and even cleaned up after we ate. We had grilled chicken, hamburgers, hot dogs, corn on the cob, green beans, salad, baked beans, and plenty of other foods. I even contributed to the meal/appetizers by having my favorite green apple salsa and a black bean watermelon salsa. It was yummilicious.

The highlight of the party seemed to be the candy buffet that my "sister" Ronnall made for me. She really isn't my sister, but we grew up together as such because my dad and her mom dated each other for years. The candy buffet was beautifully decorated with the color scheme of pink, white and black. She created the buffet with all of my favorite candies. However, it seemed as though my favorite candies were everyone else's favorites, too. By the end of the party, there was hardly any candy left.

Even though the purpose of the party was to celebrate my life, I decided to share it with other breast cancer survivors. I believe there were four of us there at the party. I bought a cake that had "Breast Cancer Survivors" inscribed on it. I also bought pink SURVIVOR bracelets, which I gave to the other survivors.

About one hundred and fifty people came to celebrate with me. I had such a great time. I think I went to bed with a smile on my face for the two nights after my party. Thank you everyone for coming out and sharing in my celebration. I love you all.

I've been so consumed with planning my party that I never got a chance to let you all know where I'm in the reconstruction process. Currently, I am still getting expanded. I really dread the days I have to get expanded, but fortunately they are coming to an end soon. I'm hoping tomorrow's appointment is the last one before my next surgery. I'm trying not to get overly anxious, or even frustrated because it seems like this process is taking forever. I am thankful for life!!! I have to keep that in mind. I can't believe I've been going through this for ten months now.

WEDNESDAY, AUGUST 25, 2010 5:01 PM; 321 days since my diagnosis; 4 minutes since last post

Just as a reminder, we are a little over two weeks away for the Race for the Cure. I received my t-shirt and bib earlier this week. I am getting excited about this walk. For those of you who may not know, I was chosen to speak at the Survivor's Ceremony prior to *the race. I am psyched. However, I have even better news. I have a date for my next surgery.*

It will take place Wednesday, October 20th. My doctor is saying I may have to be off work for three weeks. Hopefully, it won't take me that long to recuperate. I know what you're thinking, or at least what I'm thinking, October 20th is pretty far away. Yes, kind of, but I'm glad that I finally have a date. I've been waiting to receive authorization from my insurance and now I finally have it. I am finally seeing the light at the end of the tunnel.

SUNDAY, SEPTEMBER 12, 2010 3:00 PM; 338 *days since my diagnosis.*

It's the day after the Race for the Cure and I'm still in awe. Even though I've done these walks before, yesterday was amazing. The weather was perfect, my family and friends were in attendance, and I was able to complete the course. My day started around 7:30 a.m. since I had to check-in early in preparation for me giving my inspirational message to survivors. The Survivor's Ceremony was scheduled to start around 8:00 a.m.

Prior to the ceremony, all of the survivors met up and were separated in groups based on the number of years of survival, 25+ years all the way down to less than 1 year. I was in the less than 1 year group. Some of the people in my group were still going through chemo, without hair, weak, etc. They were warriors. I tell you, I am just happy to have that part of my life behind me. But at least I was able to be an example of where they'll be in a few months. We shared our stories about chemo, radiation, fake boobs, etc. It really was great talking to others who understood.

When it was time to walk out into the arena, they started with the longest survivors (25+ years) which meant my group was the last to enter through the tunnel. It was overwhelming seeing all the people in the stands cheering for us. I became a little emotional and teary-eyed just before we entered the arena, but I was able to regroup. However, once I saw the "A" Team in the stands, I began to cry...just a little. I couldn't allow myself to get too emotional because I had to deliver my speech.

Since I was representing the "Newly Diagnosed" group, I was one of the first survivors to speak. I tried to make sure I didn't speak too fast. I'll see how it went once I get the video. For those who are curious *as to what my message was, it was supposed to go as follows:*

"Good morning! My name is Andrea Campbell and I'm from Cleveland, OH. I was recently diagnosed with breast cancer. Today, my words of inspiration to you are as follows: No one knows the challenge better than you. Advice is fine, but trust your own instincts and follow your heart. With that being said, keep on keeping on, little by little, one day at a time."

I thought I had memorized the words so I wouldn't have to read from the note card, but somewhere in the middle I kind of forgot what I was supposed to say. I began to improvise. I was able to get the same point across, just with different words. The person who was in charge said I was great, so I'll receive that. After the speech, I was presented with a beautiful bouquet of flowers from the organizers of the ceremony.

This was my first time even attending the Survivor's Ceremony. Being able to have it inside of an arena was great. I was able to see everyone marching in and there were seats for everyone else to participate, too. Also, with it being indoors with seats, my 93.9-year-old grandmother was able to participate.

After the ceremony, the "A" Team met up for a group photo. (A special shout-out to my sorority sister for taking the picture). There were almost forty people who participated in the "A" Team. After the picture, it was time to walk. Three point one miles, here we come. Some of us casually walked and some of us, well, some walked much faster. I think it took me about one and a half hours to finish the 3.1 miles. I actually started behind the first group because there were so many people out there. It was a fun time and shout out to Anton (Jackie's husband) for holding the "A" Team sign during the entire walk. Also, I must send out a special thank you to my cousin/niece/daughter Ms. Teryn for decorating my sign.

I am so appreciative of everyone that participated yesterday and for those who supported me financially. I have already exceeded my goal of $1,500. The "A" Team is near $1,900, but I'm continuing to accept donations online until October 10th. If you would like, you can still donate to the "A" Team.

I also want to thank those of you whom I don't know personally, but who have prayed for me, supported my family and friends, and/or donated to the cause.

Well, I guess that's it for now. October 20th is the

next big day and I'm so ready for it to come. Goodbye for now…

Oh, I almost forgot to mention this. Yesterday, I walked in celebration of all who have survived breast cancer. I didn't get a chance to write their names on my back, but with each step, I was honoring us.

I also walked in memory of someone who lost her life due to breast cancer. It just so happened that the night before the race, I was shopping at TJ Maxx. I was being one of those rude patrons who was talking to my uncle on the telephone while I was checking out. He and I were talking about the race and I mentioned I needed to go home and prepare for my speech.

The cashier said, "I don't mean to be listening to your conversation, but are you speaking at the Race for the Cure event tomorrow?"

I said, "Yes, I am speaking at the Survivor's Ceremony."

"So you're a survivor?"

I enthusiastically said, "Yes I am!"

She proceeded to tell me she had lost her mom to breast cancer. My heart dropped. I told her I was sorry to hear about her mom and asked if she was planning to come tomorrow. She mentioned that she and her sister had thought about it, but it was too soon and, still too emotional for them right now. I told her I understood, but I would be looking for her to be there next year to honor her mom. I left the store, but as I as walked to my car, I felt like I needed to do more. I thought to myself, "I can walk in honor of her mom."

I went back into the store and asked her for her mom's name, birth date, and the day she passed away. Her mom had passed away just under a month ago on August 17th. The young lady told me that this was her mother's second battle with breast cancer. At the time of her death, she was only 44 years old with four children. I encouraged the young lady/teenager to stay on top of her health, especially since her mom passed at such a young age.

It hurts my heart to hear this story because too many women are dying. I will continue to praise God for my life. I know it's only because of his grace that I'm here. We have to find a cure...soon. Unless things change, one out of eight women will be affected with breast cancer. That's too many of us.

SUNDAY, OCTOBER 10, 2010 10:14 AM; 366 days since my diagnosis.

Last Friday marked a year since I heard the words, "You have breast cancer." I can remember it like it was yesterday. What a year! This experience seems surreal. Here I am a year later and cancer-free. This is a blessing. However, it's crazy that I am still going through the process.

My next surgery is scheduled ten days from now and that day can't come soon enough. I'm so ready to put all this behind me and to get these brick hard expanders out of me. They are so hard and painful at times. I still don't sleep well because of them...and these hot flashes. I've gone from being the lover of ninety degrees' temperature, to now wanting to roll down the window in my car when it's forty degrees outside. My doctor said that these flashes will go away eventually, but it's taking longer than I would like. Anyway, I'll be back to share with you all next week before my surgery. Until then, I love you and God bless.

TUESDAY, OCTOBER 19, 2010 2:22 PM; 375 days since my diagnosis.

Tomorrow is the day I get my new boobs. I want to ask for your continued prayers as I have my surgery. It is scheduled to take place tomorrow at 2:20

p.m. I am going to be good and hungry by then. Once I'm feeling up to it, I will give you the update as to how things go.

THURSDAY, OCTOBER 21, 2010 3:04 AM; 377 days since my diagnosis.

Hello all. This will be quick. I want to let you know that I'm back home recuperating after my surgery. Everything went well yesterday, although my surgery didn't start until 5:00 p.m. It was a long day of waiting and as you can imagine, I was very hungry. I'll give you a little more details tomorrow if I feel up to it.

TUESDAY, NOVEMBER 16, 2010 9:24 PM; 403 days since my diagnosis.

I can't believe it's been almost a month since I've blogged. I hope you all didn't miss me much. The last time I wrote, I said I would continue my story the next day, if I felt up to it. Honestly, I just didn't feel like writing. It wasn't that I didn't have anything to say, because you know I can find something to say. I needed some time away from this...whatever this is. The surgery was a success and I actually healed relatively well. Physically, the boobs did good. The main issues that I had were with my strength and endurance. I tired easily. Fortunately, I'm doing much better now. I have resumed my workout regimen. Okay, okay, okay. I've walked on my treadmill for the past three days...baby steps.

As surreal as the experience has been, I can't believe I'm done with everything. I still shake my head thinking back to all that I've been through. But God. That's all I can say. This past year was challenging to say the least, and I need a mental break.

In the next few weeks, I will be treating myself to a vacation. I just need some time to relax, reflect, and experience a new beginning. In case you want to know, I will be going to Costa Rica. Yippie.

Even though all my treatments and surgeries are completed, there is still some healing that needs to take place. I still suffer from chemo brain, but my doctor says it'll get better with time. I always joke that I used to be really, really, really smart, but now I'm just smart. And yes, this takes some getting used to, but I know I'll be back to my old self soon enough. If not, then I'll just have to adapt to the "new" me.

As I reflect on the past year, I get emotional. As I always say, I can't believe that this is my life. However, all the love and support that you all gave me was incredible. I know I say this all the time, *but you guys are amazing. The calls, cards, prayers, thoughts, everything was so appreciated. To be this loved and to know it and feel it is absolutely awesome. I couldn't end my journaling without taking the time to thank you all again. I love y'all more than you know.*

I planned to close down my account after this last entry, but someone mentioned to me recently they had given someone instructions so they can get on my site. This person is starting her journey with cancer. So, I'll keep it up a while longer and touch base periodically. I'm glad my site can encourage others in their own personal struggles. I know of at least one person this site has helped, and for that I'm grateful. In fulfilling my life's purpose, I have to realize that my testimony isn't to be kept to myself. I must share it with as many people as I can...and as you all know, I have. There are not too many women I meet that I haven't told they need to feel their boobs. I was caught off guard with this disease, but now I know that early detection is key and I'll keep preaching that for the rest of my life until a cure is found.

I am more than a conqueror!

[personal reflection]

I was overjoyed to be done with everything. It was a heck of a journey. I can now put this behind me and move forward. Now that I've completed the reconstruction process, this is a good place for me to stop and talk about life after breast cancer. Of course I am relieved all of my surgeries were successful and I'm cancer-free, however there are other changes I have to come to grip with post-surgery. My physical body has been altered permanently. My original boobs are gone. With everything that has been going on with my cancer battle, I really haven't had time to reflect on how my psyche would accept the "new" me. How will I feel about being a woman without "real" boobs? I know I have my implants, my "fake" boobs, which will stay lifted for eternity, but it isn't the same as having the boobs that I watched grow (slowly) from puberty. No, they weren't the biggest, actually they weren't big at all, but they were mine. Fortunately, my boobs didn't define me. I have come to accept that my original ones are gone and what I have now is a reminder of God's grace. Keeping my boobs was not worth risking the chance of a reoccurrence, so I'm totally at peace with the decision I made. Even though I wasn't sure how my sexuality would be affected after the loss of my boobs, I can honestly say I still feel like a woman. My boobs (and/or lack thereof) don't define my femininity.

Once I finished my treatments and surgeries, I felt the need to decompress. What better way to do that than to go on a vacation? Not just any vacation, but one where I could relax and put my toes in the sand. As I mentioned in the blog, I went to Costa Rica. Initially, I was going to visit the San Jose area of Costa Rica which is closer to the Caribbean Sea, however I decided to vacation on the Pacific Ocean side, in the Guanacaste area.

This was the most amazing vacation ever. I traveled there during the beginning of December, which is right after their rainy season. Everything was so lush and beautiful. I stayed at the JW Marriott resort, in a room with an amazing ocean view. I was able to see the sunset every day from the comfort of my room if I chose to. The resort had everything I needed. A beach, bar, and food. I didn't have to leave the resort to have a great time. However, I met a couple of people from Washington D.C. who just happened to own property in Costa Rica. They were both authors who fell in love with Costa Rica during one of their visits. They spend half of the year in D.C. and the other half in Costa Rica. The only negative thing they mentioned about living there was that the water didn't get hot at their property (and in most places in Costa Rica). They were staying at the resort for a couple of weeks just to enjoy hot water.

It was great hanging out with fellow Americans. They had a car, so I was able to leave the JW Marriott property and explore the town with them. We went to a "Christmas is Coming" festival where they had bulls running around. It's not the running of the bulls like you see in the streets of Spain, but they had bulls enclosed in a stadium and anyone could just go run around (and away) from them. It was fun to watch, especially when it looked as though the bull was going to...well you know how it goes. Feliz Navidad.

Also, I spent some of my time horseback riding on the property, zip lining through the jungles, and touring the volcano. I went to the hot springs and decompressed. It was a great time and great adventure. This was just what I needed. I left that country with the biggest smile on my face. Did I mention that Costa Rica is considered the happiest place in the world to live? After visiting there, I can understand why. Pura Vida.

———————

FRIDAY, MARCH 4, 2011 9:04 AM; 511 days since my diagnosis.

HAPPY NEW YEAR! I know I'm really late, but I haven't been on the site for a while. Even though I am approaching one year of being cancer-

free, there is one more surgery that I must endure. This afternoon, I will have my last breast reconstruction surgery. The plastic surgeon is going to perform nipple reconstruction on both breasts that should closely match my previous ones...at least I hope so. You may be wondering how the plastic surgeon will do that. I had the same thought. What I've learned is that basically he will cut the skin on the breast and make a flap which would be used to create the nipple. He will use fat from the area around my breast to rebuild the nipple.

Even after he explained the procedure to me, I still couldn't picture exactly how he was going to create the nipple. I decided to see if there were any videos of the procedure on YouTube. Wouldn't you know it? There are numerous videos that show how to create a nipple post mastectomy. It is a work of art creating the nipples. If you're curious about the procedure, you can look it up on the Internet.

I'm so ecstatic this will be my final surgery in this breast cancer journey. I am asking for your prayers today. I'm almost finished for real this time. I can finally put this behind me and move on.

TUESDAY, APRIL 12, 2011 9:28 AM; *550 days since my diagnosis.*

Today, I celebrate one year of being cancer-free. I am so grateful to God for keeping His promise to give me hope and a future. At times, I still can't believe this is my life, yet I still shake my head in awe of God. I thank Him for His love and His grace, His amazing grace. Also, I am thankful for the joy He puts in my heart every morning. *Singing loudly in my alto voice*

"Jesus, You're the center of my joy. All that's good and perfect comes from You. You're the heart of my contentment, hope for all I do. Jesus, You're the center of my joy." [4]

Thank you Richard Smallwood for those words.

Earlier this week, I received a random email that said, "You block your dreams when you allow your fear to grow bigger than your faith." – Mary Morissey. These words came right on time because I remember when I was first diagnosed with breast cancer back in 2009, I couldn't/wouldn't allow myself to be afraid. No, it wasn't a battle I wanted to fight. No, I didn't know what to expect. However, I knew that God didn't give us the spirit of fear and that I needed to put my trust in Him and His word. So, I ask the question, "Is your fear bigger than your faith?" It makes you think, huh? There is no place for fear in our lives. We have to trust that God will take care of us regardless of whatever we're going through. Fear, don't try to get comfortable in my life because you are not welcomed here.

WEDNESDAY, APRIL 27, 2011 11:18 PM; *565 days since my diagnosis.*

Over the past two weeks, I had a high school classmate pass away as well as the wife of a classmate from college. This really hit home because both of these women were young. One died from sickle cell anemia and the other died from breast cancer. Even though I hadn't seen the one from my high school in years, I was still affected by her death caused by breast cancer. I realized it could've been me. It was a reminder for me to be more diligent in getting out the message about performing monthly breast exams and having an annual mammogram. I challenge you all to continue to feel your breasts and get to know them so you will be aware of any changes that may occur. Early detection is the key to surviving breast cancer. Please pass that message along to every

woman you know. Even the men need to check themselves, too.

Now that I've delivered my public service
announcement, I'm on to the other reason I'm journaling tonight. I'm not sure why I'm being led to
say this, but I just feel that I should. Back when I
was diagnosed with breast cancer, I was full of emotions. I can't even describe every emotion that I felt
at the moment. I was scared. I was sad. Even though
I believed I was going to be victorious in this battle, I
knew that it was all God's will and I had to prepare
myself mentally for whatever. I just thank God for
His love, grace and mercy because I would be...well,
I would be dead without it.

I remember having to tell my family and my
friends. It was very difficult to say those words. After
a while, I let folk find out by word of mouth. It was
hard to keep talking about it all the time, which is
why I began blogging. I remember when I wrote my
first blog, I welcomed people to share their words of
encouragement. I welcomed phone calls, too. Anything just to let me know I was not in this journey by
myself and I was going to be okay. There were some
folk that I was disappointed in because they never
contacted me via this blog, phone, text message, or

mail. Nothing. I knew in my heart that they were concerned because they would ask other people about me, but they never reached out to me to see how I was doing.

When I would bring it to their attention, they would say they didn't know what to say or they didn't know how to handle the situation. Let me just say, I'm not talking about one person in particular so please don't get offended if you feel as though I'm talking about you. I need to let people know that my feelings were hurt. I know some folk think they don't know what to say in these situations or even how to express what they feel. I mean, what if I would have died? Would they have been okay knowing they never told me what they were thinking about me or that they even cared? Couldn't they have called to say that they're praying for me? Or just say hello? Keep in mind, I'm saying this in love. Most of the people I'm talking about probably won't even see this journal update.

This situation reminds me of my friend, Valaria, who sat next to me in the choir. Over time, we developed a close friendship. Six years ago, she was diagnosed with cancer. I can't remember which kind of cancer, but she ended up in hospice care during her last days. My feelings were hurt when I found out.

I remember thinking to myself, "I don't want to go see her like that. I don't want to have anything to do with cancer. I'm still not over my sister's death from cancer."

Mentally, I wasn't ready to see her like that nor deal with the reality of the situation. She was fighting for her life, just as I had seen my sister do some years before.

Then one day I heard that she only had a few days to live. My heart was broken. I hadn't seen her yet and now I was faced with a dilemma. Either I had to go see her in in hospice or I would see her at her funeral. I finally made my way to her bedside. When I walked into her room, the first thing she said to me was, "It's about time. I've been waiting for you to come see me."

I began to cry immediately.

Surprisingly, when I saw her, she didn't look like I thought she would. She was in great spirits. She was at peace with everything that was going on. I explained to her why it took me so long to come see her, and in that moment, I realized how selfish I had been. This wasn't about me. She was fighting for her life and I couldn't even get over myself (and my issues) to go see her, pray with her, or even let her know that I cared. I still shake my head in disappointment of myself because who knew she would be me some years later...kinda.

Unfortunately, she'll never know the lesson she taught me, but I felt the need to share it with you all. Sometimes we have to put others' needs first before our own selfishness. It ain't always about me/us (...and yes, I know that's bad grammar). It wouldn't have killed me to go visit her sooner. I'm thankful that I was able to see her and tell her how I felt about her before she died.

Yes, it was uncomfortable for me to go see her, and yes it brought up some feelings that I wasn't ready to deal with, but really, was that more important than letting her know that I cared? Life is short, too short. We do not know when our last breath will be, so as long as we have it, we need make sure that we let those we care about know how we feel, regardless of how uncomfortable it makes us feel.

Like I said before, I'm just saying this in love. Maybe it'll get someone thinking about their situation and how they need to get over themselves, too. Who knows?

Well, if nothing else, I feel better now. I'm not sure why this was placed on my heart, but it needed to be said because it has been there for a little while.

P.S. It's kind of late so I hope this reads easily because I'm cross-eyed right now.

[personal reflection]

This public service announcement was heavy on my heart. I had been carrying that load of shame and guilt for some time. Who knew that I would be in a similar situation? As I mentioned above, I was taught an invaluable lesson by my friend, Valaria. It's one that I needed to share. Because of my past experiences, I was trying to protect myself from hurt and pain. I hadn't even thought about the hurt and pain my friend was experiencing. Initially, I wasn't willing to sacrifice my own uncomfortableness to make someone else comfortable. Sometimes, we get so caught up in ourselves and our individual lives that we forget that we're all connected. I need you. You need me. We all need each other to survive.

This is a lesson that I will carry with me forever. It was life-changing for me and I hope it gives you another perspective to consider the next time you're trying to avoid being uncomfortable.

Reflection Questions

1. *Can you think of a situation you're dealing with where you need to get over yourself?*
2. *Are you willing to make yourself uncomfortable to help make someone else comfortable?*
3. *What are you willing to sacrifice to help someone else who's in need?*

16

what the what?!?

"I AM NOT AFRAID OF STORMS FOR I AM LEARNING
HOW TO SAIL MY SHIP."

– LOUISA MAY ALCOTT

———

I know, I know, I know. I hear it all the time. "You do
not look like someone who has gone through cancer." But what does someone who has gone through
cancer look like? I must admit I look amazing. My
skin is smooth and it's glowing. I just say it's God's
grace radiating through me. Looks can be deceiving,

huh? It's hard to look at someone and truly know what they are going through or even what they've been through. Recently, I have been listening to the song "Life and Favor" by John P. Kee. It has been on repeat for the past couple of weeks. I will share some of the words of this song because it's easy to make judgments about people based on what you see, but you don't know their story...

You don't know my story
You don't know the things that I've come through
You cannot imagine
The pain the trials I've had to endure...
In all God has been faithful to me
He promised He would never leave me
My story proves that God can use me
Deliverance is my testimony
You don't know — my story... [5]

We **ALL** have a story to tell. I can't look at you and assume I know how life has treated you. You can walk through this world and look as though everything is great, yet you're dying on inside. We must be mindful of how we treat people because we don't know what they have gone through, or what they are currently going through. All of us have experienced adversity that has challenged us. We've all experienced hurt, trials and tribulations, but the hope is that we'll come out of these situations better than we were before. *God never wastes a hurt.*

Romans 8:28 (KJV) says, "And we know that all things work together for good to them that love God, to them who are called according to his purpose." Everything that we go through is for our good, if we trust and believe in His word. It helps mold us into the unique beings that we are meant to be.

Cancer didn't slow me down nor did I use it as an excuse to give up on life. Honestly, I look at my breast cancer diagnosis as a blessing. I know that may sound strange, but it's true. It forced me to slow down and take some time to look at Andrea; to look at the person I was and help create the person I wanted to be. Even though the roads to becoming cancer-free weren't easy, they were necessary. The old me had to go. I have morphed into a better me. One who's more compassionate. One who's wiser. One who's stronger. One who's less judgmental. One who lives intentionally and purposefully. So yes, cancer was a blessing for me. This journey has given me so many grand ideas as to how I want to positively impact the world. I can't wait to see what the universe has to offer next.

Since my battle with cancer, I have been intentional about creating great memories. In July 2011, I had my Celebration of Life, Part Deux party. Just like the year before, it was a blast. I had great food, great music, and great fellowship. The weather was perfect and once the party was over outside, we brought it inside to my basement. We played games, continued to eat, and sang karaoke. I appreciated all the love and support that was given to me.

My brother and niece came to town to celebrate with me and brought my great-nephew, Elijah to Cleveland for his two-week visit with me. I love this little guy and he loves his auntie right back. He was 6 years old and I thought it would be great to surprise him and take him to Disney World. I knew we would have so much fun.

However, instead of my brother and niece just bringing Elijah, they brought one of my other nephews, Donald. He rode to Cleveland with them to visit for the weekend. I hadn't shared with anyone my plans for Disney. I was the only person who had known of the surprise I had planned for Elijah.

I started feeling guilty knowing that my brother and niece were planning to take my other nephew back with them and I was about to take Elijah on his first plane ride to an amazing destination. I knew Donald would love to go, too. Fortunately, I had rented a place in Florida that had two bedrooms, so having a place for him to sleep wouldn't be a deterrent for me having him to come with us. I needed to make sure I could find him a seat on our flight. It wouldn't do me any good to ask him if he wanted to go if I couldn't get another seat on the plane.

Now mind you, this was three days before departure, so as you can imagine, flights weren't inexpensive. Fortunately, I was able to get him a seat at the last minute using my airline points. I asked Donald if he wanted to stay in Cleveland for a couple of weeks and, of course he said yes. He had only brought enough clothes for two days, so not only did I have to take him clothes shopping, but also, I had to enroll him in summer camp like I had done for Elijah. Those were just some of the technicalities that I needed to work out.

So now, I was taking my two nephews to Disney. The day before our trip, I surprised both of the boys by letting them in on it. "We are going to Disney!" They were happy, but not as excited as I was for them. I knew we were going to have a good time and this was going to be a great experience for both of them. It happened that my best friend, Jackie, her husband, Anton and the Raggedies were going to be at Disney World during the same time we were there. This allowed us to take in some of the Disney experience together.

This was the first time on an airplane for both of

my nephews. They really enjoyed the experience of flying. Once we arrived in Orlando, we went to the rental agency to pick up my car. I surprised the boys by renting a candy apple red Mustang. When they saw the car, they were über excited. At that moment, I was the coolest auntie ever. We got in the car and drove to the resort to get ourselves situated.

The resort was very nice and clean. There was a pond with a water fountain shooting up from the middle of it. The boys were fascinated with it because there were ducks swimming around in it. Once we arrived to our suite, I was even more impressed with the resort. Our suite consisted of two bedrooms, two bathrooms, a kitchen, a dining room, and a living room. The boys were staying on the opposite side of the suite and we didn't have to share a bathroom. Anyone who has lived with boys know that was a huge bonus.

Later that afternoon, we met up with Jackie and her family so we could head to the water park together. The kids really enjoyed themselves there. Afterward, we went to McDonalds where the kids ate and played games. After realizing how much money we spent on food the first day, we decided to go grocery shopping to buy food for breakfast and lunch. By having a kitchen in my suite, we able to save money because we didn't have to pay to eat out for every meal. Anton cooked breakfast in the mornings and we would pack our lunch for the park.

On our second day in Orlando, we went to the Epcot theme park. The highlight was when we went Soarin'. Soarin' is a flight simulator attraction that lifts its guests on multi-passenger hang gliders for a scenic aerial tour of California. If you've ever experienced Soarin', then you know how much fun it is. If you haven't, it's a must the next time you visit Epcot.

The kids had a blast. Disney World had proven to really be the happiest place in the world...at least for the kids. For me, on the other hand, it was the most expensive place. I was going broke from spending all my money on the theme parks and food for dinner. The ironic thing is that the kids' favorite part of the trip was playing in the pool at the resort. Had I known that was going to be the case, I could've saved a lot of money and played in a pool back in Cleveland. At least now I know better. However, I hope they will come to appreciate the trip and their auntie when they get older.

The day before we were to leave Orlando, I began feeling horrible. I woke up having indescribable, excruciating abdominal pains. I called Jackie to see if she and Anton could entertain the boys while I tried to get myself together. They kept the boys with them until they had to leave for the airport to catch their flight back to Cleveland.

Once they left, it was just me and the boys. Fortunately, I was feeling much better by this time. We had one more day at Disney and I was determined to make the most of it. That evening, we went to Magic Kingdom where we rode the thrill rides, celebrated with the Disney characters in the parade, and watched the fireworks.

The next morning, we woke up early so that we could visit the Animal Kingdom theme park before we left Orlando. We had such a great time while we were there. Elijah and Donald loved having up-close encounters with the animals and I was still feeling pretty good.

After the park, we headed back to the airport to catch our flight. First, I had to drop off the rental car. As I drove to the rental agency, I began having the same pains as the day before. I tried to pretend as though everything was okay with me since I had the boys, but it wasn't. I didn't know the cause of my pain, but I knew something was wrong. I needed to get home quickly. I needed to hurry up and get back to Cleveland so that I could see the doctor to find out what was going on with me.

Just before it was time for us to board our flight, my pain became worse (as if that was even possible).

I told the boys to stay in their seats and proceeded to run to the restroom. While I was in there, all I could do was call on the name of Jesus. The pain was intense. Very intense. I needed to get back home, but I couldn't even get myself to the plane. I began to cry.

While I was in the bathroom stall crying, I looked over at the floor of the stall next to me. All I could see was someone's feet. All of a sudden, a feeling of confusion came over me. *"Why are...why are those shoes facing the wrong way?"*

It was at that moment when I realized I was in the wrong place. In my haste, I ran into the first restroom I saw, which happened to be the men's restroom. Oh My Goodness! I couldn't even laugh at myself because I was in such severe pain.

After peeking underneath and seeing all the shoes were gone, I ran out of the stall, out of the restroom, got my boys, and boarded the plane.

I was still having pain and I knew in my heart that something was terribly wrong. I sat in my seat crying the entire flight home. I bought each of the boys their own movies so I didn't have to hear them argue over what to watch. They didn't even notice I was crying the entire time.

All these thoughts crossed my mind. What *can this be? What is going on with me? What is causing all this pain? Something isn't right. I need to make an appointment with my doctor first thing in the morning.*

We had traveled two and one-half hours before we began our final descent into Cleveland. The boys hadn't paid me any mind on the flight as they watched their respective movies in peace. The flight attendant announced that we would be landing soon so to make sure our seat belts were fastened, the seats were in the upright position, and our tray tables were up. We were almost back in Cleveland and I was so ready to get off this plane so I could get home.

It was at this point when my nephews noticed my tears. They asked me what was wrong and I began to cry even harder. That's when Donald mentioned he needed to go to the restroom. What? We had been on this flight for over two hours and he waited until he couldn't get up out of his seat to tell me he needs to go to the restroom. I told him he had to hold it until we got off the plane.

The plane landed. Fortunately, we were near the front of the plane, so we would be one of the first to get off. When we finally got off, we sprinted to the restrooms. The situation was a mess...*literally.*

I was able to drive home even though I was in excruciating pain. I knew that if I could get home to my prescription medication, I would be fine.

Once we arrived home, I took one of the pain pills. Nothing. It didn't even begin to touch the pain, not one bit. I was too scared to take another, so I decided it would be best to go to the Emergency Room. As private as I am, I didn't want anyone to have to worry about me, especially since I didn't know what was wrong. I really didn't want to tell my mom, however I needed somebody to watch the boys while I went to the ER. I called my mom and told her about my situation. She came to pick up my nephews.

My childhood friend, Cassandra, called me as I was driving to the hospital. I told her what was going on and she met me at the Emergency Room. She waited with me until I was able to see the doctor. When I saw the ER physician, he examined me and said it looked like I had some fibroid tumors that were causing the pain. Fibroid tumors are non-cancerous growths of the uterus that often appear during childbearing years. They are common in African American women. The ER physician suggested that I see my GYN physician as soon as possible.

I know this may be (or become) TMI for some. Sorry, but again I'm only sharing for informational purposes. Feel free to skip down to the next blog if you like. I'm want to be as transparent as I can so I can possibly help someone, anyone. We never know how one's mess, can turn into a message, which in turn can save a life. It's not easy sharing this because it takes me back to a place I really don't want to go. Nonetheless, I will continue with the story.

After I left the ER, I made an appointment with a random GYN, someone who I had never seen before. I needed to get in right away and at this point, I didn't care who I saw. Thank goodness for electronic medical records because the doctors were able to review my medical history.

Over the next few days, I met with doctors, had examinations, and biopsies performed. The doctors recommended a hysterectomy because the fibroids were so large that they didn't know if my uterus would be of use. The fibroid had taken up so much space that it would be difficult for a baby to grow in it.

Of course, having a hysterectomy wasn't what I wanted to do. Heck, I had gone through the egg harvesting process to give myself a chance for a baby. Now they wanted me to have a hysterectomy? After much conversation and prayer, I decided to only have the fibroids removed and keep my uterus intact. I was aware I had fibroid tumors, but they hadn't really bothered me much before. Now, I needed them gone as soon as possible because they were causing me unbearable pain. I was scheduled to have surgery on July 28th.

On the morning of surgery, Jackie came to pick me up and we headed to the hospital. While in route, I received a telephone call.

"Hello."

"Is this Andrea?"

"Yes it is. Who's calling?"

"This is Dr. Z. I know you are scheduled for surgery in a couple of hours, but I just received the results from your biopsy."

"Uh huh."

"I'm sorry to tell you this, but the biopsy came back positive for cancer."

WAIT, WHAT? WHAT THE WHAT? YOU'VE GOT TO BE KIDDING ME! I DID NOT SEE THIS COMING AT ALL. THIS CANNOT BE MY LIFE! IT JUST CAN'T BE...

I didn't even have a chance to say anything to Jackie before she asked, "Is it cancer again?"

I began to cry.

Reflection Question

1. *How do you handle life's challenges when they seem to keep knocking you down?*

17

here we go again...

"I LEARNED THAT LIFE WILL GO THROUGH CHANGES —
UP AND DOWN AND UP AGAIN. IT'S WHAT LIFE DOES."

— BEN OKRI

THURSDAY, JULY 28, 2011 10:04 PM; 657 *days
since my* 1st *diagnosis.*

Today, July 28, 2011 has to be the second worst
day of my life. I have to trust God through all of
this. "For I know the plans I have for you, declares
the Lord, plans to prosper you and not to harm you,

plans to give you a hope and a future." – Jeremiah 29:11. Here we go again...

[a quick reflection]

I can't believe this was my life again. As you can see by this post, I couldn't even bring myself to talk about it yet. Fortunately, Jackie was with me when I found out about the cancer because I couldn't even think straight. After hearing my diagnosis, Jackie turned the car around and we headed back to my house. She said that we needed to figure out how to get my mom to my house without alarming her to my situation. My mom was supposed to be meeting us at the hospital in a few minutes.

I was still in shock. Jackie had me call my friend, Q so he could come back to my house. He had stopped by earlier to pray with me before surgery. Throughout all of this mess, he had been right there with me and had been a great supporter, even before I/we knew how serious this "mess" was. Once he arrived, I told him what was going on and he assured me everything would be fine.

When my mom finally made it to my house, it was deja vu. Once again, I couldn't put the words together to tell my mom I had cancer. Jackie had to tell her, even though I think she suspected it. She took the news better than I thought she would. I am so grateful for my support system. I wouldn't have made it through without them.

Understandably, I was upset after this diagnosis. Not just for me having to go through it again, but also for those who supported me the first time. They had to go through this again, too. I didn't do a lot of calling to share the news. I let everyone else do it for me this time. I didn't want to have to talk about it. Plus, I was still in pain. After a few days, I decided I needed to let those who follow me on my blog know about my situation. This was going to be a shock to some folk. I was sorry to have to do this to them again, but I needed prayers to go up.

I found myself confused by this diagnosis. I didn't even know how to pray to God this time. I was mad at Him. Why would He allow this to happen again, especially in such a short amount of time? Although I couldn't answer that question, I knew I had to just trust Him again. I may never know why I had to go through this again, but it's all for my good, right?

Things moved quicker this time around. After talking to the GYN oncologist, my surgery was scheduled for the following Wednesday. It just happened to be on the same day as the concert I was supposed to attend featuring Jill Scott and Anthony Hamilton. Yes, I was petty enough to ask my doctor if he could postpone the surgery for one more day so I could make the concert. I mean, I had already bought my ticket to see them and I absolutely love Jill Scott. As you can probably guess, I missed the concert.

MONDAY, AUGUST 1, 2011 12:32 PM; *661 days since my 1st diagnosis; 4 days since my 2nd diagnosis.*

I can't believe I have to start counting the days all over again.

I guess I need to share with you all what is going on with me. I know it's been a while since I've blogged on this site. I only keep it up and running to keep folk informed about the Race for the Cure coming up in September. The "A" Team will still be representing, unfortunately without me.

Last week, I was diagnosed with uterine cancer. Yes, you read it correctly. I am battling cancer...again. I was not expecting this news, nor did I even suspect anything close to this. This time around, I've had severe abdominal pains. My oncologists likened the pain to that of a mother during child-birth. My uterus was trying to rid itself of the cancer by forcing it to constantly contract. Even though I have a pretty high tolerance for pain, that pain was unbearable. I apologize for sharing this news on the site, but I really needed to start updating folk so I could reduce the number of phone calls I'm receiving. Don't get me wrong, I appreciate folk checking in on me, but it is overwhelming at times.

I know this news may come as a shock to many of you, but I want everyone to be in the loop. As before, I ask for your prayers, support and words of encouragement. Surprisingly, I'm not even crying as I write this. I may be all cried out at this point or maybe I've just accepted it. I tell you, I am so not ready to have to go through this again, but it's not like I have a choice.

Right now, the doctors don't know much about the type of uterine cancer. All I know is that I am scheduled for surgery on Wednesday, August 3rd. Everything is moving much faster this time around. Once I know the time of my surgery, I will let you all know. But for now, please include me (and my family) in your thoughts and prayers.

I guess you all can now understand my last entry

and why I'm leaning so strongly on the scripture Jeremiah 29:11. I believe God's word and His promises.

WEDNESDAY, AUG 3, 2011 7:41 AM; 6 days since my 2nd diagnosis.

Surgery is today. It is scheduled for 11:00 a.m. Please keep me in your prayers.

THURSDAY, AUGUST 4, 2011 1:01 PM; 7 days since my 2nd diagnosis.

My surgery went well yesterday and I'm just recuperating slowly. It's very painful, but hopefully the pain won't last too long...who am I kidding? It's gonna be a long, slow recovery.

TUESDAY, AUGUST 9, 2011 11:25 AM; 12 days since my 2nd diagnosis.

I just want to let everyone know that I'm back home recovering. Thanks for all the prayers, thoughts and well wishes. I will get back blogging once I'm feeling a little stronger and when I have more information. Until then, take care.

WEDNESDAY, AUGUST 24, 2011 11:03 AM; 25 days since my 2nd diagnosis.

Okay, I'm back. This time, recovery has taken a little longer than before. I haven't been able to be on the computer as much. Recovery is supposed to be six to eight weeks. We'll see how things go. I'm definitely not going to push it. However, I'm doing pretty good right now. I am getting stronger each day and my spirits are still pretty good for the most part. There are moments when I sit and think to myself, "I can't believe this is my life." I know I've said this before but...

Having uterine cancer has been different from having breast cancer in the sense that I really don't have many decisions to make. It was a no-brainer that my uterus had to go along with anything else that was attached to it or in the vicinity. During surgery, I lost a lot of blood and had to have a blood transfusion.

I haven't spoken to my GYN oncologist/surgeon since I was in the hospital and my next appointment isn't until September 2nd. I don't have much information to share besides the fact that the type of the cancer I had was rare. It's called an Endometrial Stromal Sarcoma (ESS). Less than 1 percent of people will get this kind of cancer. *Shaking my head* I think I heard my doctor say that less than four hundred people in the world per year get this particular type of cancer and there's a 40 percent chance of recurrence.

I was in a state of shock as he was speaking and I haven't bothered to listen to the recording from my appointment. I haven't done much research on it yet, mainly because I don't have the energy. My psyche isn't ready just yet. One thing I do know is that this cancer is not related to my other cancer.

I'm not sure what my next steps are. I may have to do chemo again, radiation or both. I have to fully recuperate before I can start anything. As always, I'll keep you posted. I appreciate your love, prayers and thoughts. Take care and God bless.

WEDNESDAY, SEPTEMBER 7, 2011 10:24 AM; 44 *days since my 2nd diagnosis.*

I know I've been pretty limited in the information I've shared thus far, but it's only because I haven't done much research, haven't asked many questions and...well, I'm still in disbelief that this is my life. What I can share with you is the information I received last Friday from my GYN oncologist. I found out my tumor was pretty large and one out of the thirty lymph nodes they removed showed metastasis. That means that the cancer cell has traveled to my lymph node. Because of this, I have to complete five weeks of radiation (daily) and then four and one-

*half months of chemo. As you can probably assume,
I'm pretty bummed out by this news. I really do not
want to go through chemo again, but I don't have a
choice. If I do any research on this cancer, I will let
you know what I find. Right now, I'm choosing to just
trust God in this process.*

[personal reflection]

Going through this cancer was much different than
the first one. As I mentioned earlier in the book, having a double mastectomy didn't cause me to feel as
though I lost my femininity. I looked at it as though
I was trading in my boobs for life. Yes, I miss my
breasts, but fortunately, I was able to get implants.

The uterine cancer was much different. I knew
I had to have my uterus removed, however, I didn't
know that my ovaries, fallopian tubes, and anything
else "female" had to go as well. I can remember the
conversation like it was yesterday. My doctor recommended I removed all of my reproductive organs. He
said if I didn't have them removed, it would be like
"pouring gasoline on fire." Basically, what he was trying to say is it was risky to keep them because cancer
could easily spread since I already have a gynecologic

cancer. Nothing good could come from keeping my reproductive organs.

Even though it was difficult to hear, I decided to take heed to his recommendation. Everything that was female is now gone. No boobs. No uterus. No ovaries. No fallopian tubes. No nothing. Having my reproductive organs removed caused me to have to deal with other issues. Once my ovaries were removed, I was immediately thrown into menopause. My hormones have been all over the place. Now, I can't go anywhere without carrying a fan with me because of my hot flashes. Also, I have to take calcium supplements to prevent osteoporosis.

Unfortunately, having my uterus removed took away any chance of me having a child. After going through the egg freezing process with the last cancer, I don't even have a uterus to hold a child. I am saddened by the fact that my dream of carrying a child is gone forever. I've never imagined my life without being a mom. I always thought I would have five kids and seven dogs. Fortunately, I was able to have had the opportunity to briefly experience motherhood when my niece lived with me after my sister passed away.

One of my friends, who will remain nameless, always says that kids are overrated. LOL. I know she doesn't mean that most of the time, but there are times when I know she's serious. Nonetheless, I have my godchildren, nieces and nephews who make me proud and bring me so much joy. I would've love to have a daughter who I could've named Andrea, but I'm blessed to have my namesake in my Raggedy #2, India Andrea.

People continually tell me I don't have to give up my hopes of raising a child. I can always try adopting a child or even use a surrogate. We'll see what God has planned.

THURSDAY, SEPTEMBER 8, 2011 10:24 PM; 42 days since my 2nd diagnosis.

If you recall from the last time I was going through breast cancer, my Raggedies were having a difficult time with the situation. Evidently, this time is no different. I received a call from Jackie and she tells me the girls were playing with their dolls and out of the blue, Erin, one of the twins, said her doll had cancer. She said that the doll was beautiful even though she wasn't going to have any hair and she was going to be a model. You never know how children process stuff. When I first heard the story, I cried. But then I realized that's how she's dealing with it. She recognizes you can still be beautiful without hair and you can still have hope and a future after going through cancer. With this, I guess I'll leave you with Jeremiah 29:11 again.

"For I know the plans I have for you, declares
the Lord. Plans to prosper you and not harm you.
Plans to give you a hope and a future."

I'm trusting His word. I have been standing strong on this promise time and time again.

TUESDAY, SEPTEMBER 20, 2011 2:11 PM; 54 days since my 2nd diagnosis.

I'm feeling like deja vu. Here is a repost from October 25, 2009. It's amazing how some things have change, yet they are still the same. I am sharing this again so that it can get into your spirit. Just know with God, all things are possible.

With God, every day is a day to begin again – to trust and feel His love for us and know that in all of the confusion, there is a gift to be found.

With God, every day is a day to hope for the best – to believe our prayers are being heard, that good news is on its way, that anything can happen between yesterday and tomorrow.

With God, every day is a day to count our bless-ings, to remember whose children we are, and what we're capable of through a Father who cares so much.

With God, every day is a day to be made new – to forgive and heal, to do what we can, and leave the rest to God.

– Unknown

Even though I'm in this battle, I do realize that I'm not fighting it alone. I want everyone who's going through this process with me to take a moment and meditate on those words. Believe that in this crazy mess, there's a blessing.

Trust, I would love not to have to take part in this reality show, but being I have the leading role, I will do my part and put on my best performance and beat this cancer thing. Am I scared? Yes, but then I remember that God does not give us the spirit of fear. When those thoughts cross my mind, I begin to pray and believe that I will be fine.

I don't really have much more to update you all on. I will meet with the radiation oncologist next Monday, and at that point, I'll know when my treatments will begin.

SUNDAY, OCTOBER 8, 2011 12:03 PM; 2 years

since my initial diagnosis; 72 days since my 2nd diagnosis.

It has been two years since I was diagnosed with breast cancer. I can never forget that day (even if I tried) because it was my sister's birthday and two days before my dad's. For some reason, I used to always get their birthdays confused. It took me years of conscious effort to remember whose birthday was on the 8th and whose was the 10th.

After the passing of my sister, I made sure I remembered her birthday so that I could check on her children and see how they were doing on that day. Now, it'll also be remembered as the day my life changed forever. I won't say it's the worst day of my life anymore, but the day I had a new outlook on life and how precious it really is. Each day, I'm afforded new mercies, better health, and life.

I know I haven't updated you all in a while so I'll let you know what's going on with me. A couple of weeks ago, I had a consultation with the radiation oncologist and his nurse. They shared what to expect during my radiation. There was some good news and some not-so-good news. The good news is that the radiation will kill any cells (good or bad) in the pelvic region. So if there is cancer anywhere, it will be destroyed. That's about it for the good news. The not-so-good news is all the side effects that could happen and the length of time I have to go through this.

I will have to undergo numerous radiation treatments over a nine-week period. It will consist of treatments that occur five days a week for the first five weeks, a one week break, and then treatment once a week for an additional three weeks. The side effects are fatigue, skin irritation, loss of appetite, and diarrhea. I have to eat a low residual diet, i.e. no fruit, no fresh vegetables, no whole grains, and no greasy foods. This is going to be tough especially since I love to juice and blend fruits and veggies. The side effects will be gradual so they probably won't start for a couple of weeks. They will give me cream to help with the skin irritation/burns. As far as the fatigue, I will just have to take naps as necessary.

October 1st, I had an appointment to prepare for the start of my radiation treatment. I had to do a scan and simulation of my radiation treatment. The staff performed the scan to make sure I was positioned correctly so that the radiation targeted the appropriate area.

Afterward, they took this heated plastic mesh to make a mold of my abdomen/pelvic area. This purpose of the mold was to ensure I would be in the same position with each dose of radiation. Once the mold was hardened, they repeated the scan to make sure everything was fine.

Next, they put tattoos on each side of my pelvic area so they could align the beams once they did the radiation treatments. These tattoos were only dots. They also marked my stomach and thighs so they would know where to position the mold. By the time I left, I had numerous green marks and tape on me. Forgive me if this seems confusing. It was for me as well.

The radiation therapy will be given using an IMRT machine. This machine will help localize the treatment area where they want the radiation beams to go. This could possibly help reduce the side effects. I have to go back tomorrow to do my verification. I'm not sure exactly what that is, but I think it's just to verify that everything is correct with the placement. *Shrugging shoulders*

As far as my treatments, I am scheduled to begin on Tuesday, so I'm trying to eat all the fruits and raw vegetables I can before then. I will be back on the site on Tuesday to let you know how the first treatment goes.

THURSDAY, OCTOBER 13, 2011 7:14 PM; *77 days since my 2nd diagnosis.*

Radiation treatment: Sorry it's a little late coming, but I have already completed my first radiation treatment...well, now three. Everything is going well so far. As I mentioned in my last update, I went on Monday for my "verification." The purpose of that was just to make sure the positioning was correct. Everything was fine and my first treatment was on Tuesday. I thought going through this would be a little emotional for me, but I only shed one tear. The entire process took fifteen to twenty minutes to complete. As I lie on the table, the IMRT machine rotated around me as it was giving me the necessary dose. The treatment only lasts about five to ten minutes, but each day they have to take pictures first. I think I mentioned to you about the markings and tape I had on my body when I initially went for placement. Most of them are now gone. I only have the tattoos, which are permanent, and a couple of green marks so they can easily find the tattoos.

As far as me, I'm doing fine. No side effects yet. They said that if I experience any, it'll be after two and one-half to three weeks into the treatment. Hope-

fully, I'll make it through all the treatments without experiencing any side effects. Just being optimistic.

THURSDAY, NOVEMBER 17, 2011 5:06 PM; 112 *days since my 2nd diagnosis.*

In Between Radiation: As you may recall, my last update was when I had just started my first radiation sessions. Well, I'm happy to say that I completed the twenty-five sessions and now I'm waiting for phase two to begin. I made it through better than I thought I would. It was rough and yes, I did experience most of the side effects, but I made it through. Having to go to the hospital daily was a challenge in itself, but doing the treatments was challenging, too. However, I'm not going to complain about it. I'm just happy it's over.

Next week, I will begin the brachytherapy, which is a more localized radiation treatment with a higher dose than the previous ones. This is the treatment that is once a week for three weeks. I don't know what side effects to expect this time around. I will find out at my appointment on Tuesday.

Thanks for the continued prayers. I appreciate you all standing in the gap for me. You have been praying for me when I couldn't pray for myself. I still have my moments, but I know this is all for my good. I know that I've been blessed throughout all of this because things could've been worse. Much worse.

Just in case you're wondering, I am working during this time. In addition to my full-time position, I serve on the leadership board for one of our Employee Resource Groups. When I was diagnosed with cancer the first time, I continued to volunteer my time. However, after my uterine cancer diagnosis, I knew it would be best if I relinquished my leadership role and focused solely on my health.

I called one of my friends/co-workers to let him know about my diagnosis and that I was going to step down. Before I could even tell him why I was calling, he told me he and his wife were leaving the doctor's office and she had just been diagnosed with breast cancer. Even though I was dealing with my own situation, I knew I needed to share some words of encouragement.

Every time I called him to check on his wife, it seemed like the wrong time. Either she was just finishing chemotherapy, leaving her doctor's appointment, or having a bad day. However, I know it wasn't the wrong time when I called; it was all God's *time. I was able to be supportive and give them hope through my testimony.*

My friend's wife was diagnosed with cancer around August 1ˢᵗ and unfortunately, she passed away this past Saturday. Of course, I'm affected by her death. I realize that it could've been me. But God...

I'll keep you all posted with how things go with my next treatments. If I don't get back to you before the holiday, Happy Thanksgiving to you all. Enjoy the things that matter most, your family and friends.

[personal reflection]

Wow. This is really my life, huh? Cancer, Part II was tough. I was tired. Physically and emotionally. However, I am thankful for those who supported me because they are who kept me going.

One of my main supporters was my dear friend, Q. He was a very kind and caring person with such a huge heart. He was a jewel. During my diagnosis, treatments, and recovery, he had been right there with me along the way. Besides being supportive of me, he was there for my dog, Gigi. He loved Gigi and she loved him even more. He actually taught my dog how to spell. I know that sounds crazy, but it's true...well, kinda. Of course my dog couldn't spell, but she understood words that Q spelled out for her. For instance, he would spell T-R-E-A-T and my dog would run to the cabinets where her treats were kept. He would spell E-G-G and she would run to the kitchen and look at the microwave until her egg was cooked. I'm not sharing this to brag on how amazing and smart my dog is, however she is amazing and smart. She has been right there with me during both of my ordeals. But enough about Gigi. I want to focus on my friend, Q.

I remember a few months after my cancer diagnosis, Q had gone through some health challenges, too. His challenges led to other issues. I'm not going to go into specifics, but let me just say I would've rather had his issues instead of mine. I felt as though Q's situation was temporary and it could be fixed, whereas my situation was a matter of life or death. At times, I may have seemed insensitive when he complained about his situation because I didn't think it was that serious. Yes, it sucked, but heck, it wasn't something that was going to kill him. Meanwhile, I was fighting for my life for the second time in a year and one-half. I tried to use my situation to help him realize things could be much worse. But he never seemed to get it.

Then one day, I finally got it. I was looking at

his situation all wrong. I was looking at it from my narrow perspective and not his. Everyone isn't built the same. That's what makes us unique beings. Although I didn't think his cross was too heavy to bear, he did. I needed to respect that.

This lesson was eye opening for me. I learned that I cannot judge the weight of other people's crosses/burdens based on how light they may seem to me. We are all different people with varying degrees of capabilities. Just because some crosses may seem lighter than others, it doesn't negate the heaviness that the burden may cause someone. We've all heard God doesn't give us more than we can handle. He knows exactly how much each one of us can take that will cause us to bend and not break.

I am appreciative of Q for teaching me this lesson. Unfortunately, he passed away. He was an amazing human being. I am forever grateful for his friendship.

Okay, I need to take a break from this for a moment. I miss my friend and I'm tired. I hope you felt all of my emotions through this experience. They had been all over the place. It was a tough road and I'm so glad it's over.

For now, I am going to be random and move on to another topic...

———

Reflection Questions

1. *How have your life's experiences helped you to build muscle so that you can carry your cross?*
2. *What are some life lessons that you've learned from others?*

18

I am...

Going through cancer has made me hungry for life.
I was excited to experience life after cancer. God
spared my life for a reason and I was ready to make
my life count. Instead of sitting around and binge
watching TV series, I decided to take some Executive Education courses at my alma mater, Case West-

ern Reserve University. I love to learn and this was going to help me develop into a better person, a better leader.

During one of my courses, the professor shared the following quote, "I always knew I'd be somebody. Now I realize I should've been a little more specific." When I heard this quote, I had to chuckle. Mainly, because I do know I am *somebody*, but I'm not sure if I'm the *somebody* I envisioned myself being. *Who am I really?* I've been letting life define me instead of me defining/designing my life. *What happened to all of my dreams? My dreams of being a pianist? My dreams of being a pediatrician?*

While participating in a coaching course, I created a personal vision statement for myself. This exercise was very powerful because it forced me to take a look at myself and decide who I wanted to be. After creating this vision statement, I realized I had to live my life more deliberately and more unapologetically. That exercise gave me a freedom I didn't know existed. I can design my life the way I want it to be. It's not too late. It requires me to be intentional in my words, thoughts, and actions. I want to live a life that leaves an imprint on the world and now I will be intentional about doing so.

I remember receiving a call from a friend of mine.

She and I became friends when she became my Mary Kay consultant and I sold her her first home. She asked if I would be willing to speak at her church in October, which is breast cancer awareness month. Initially, I was somewhat hesitant. I know this may come to a surprise to those who know me, but I don't necessarily like to be the center of attention. However, I believe it is my responsibility to share my story with the hope I could impact someone's life. I didn't ask for specifics at that time, but I committed to speak anyway.

Typically, at my church when we have guests come in and speak on various topics, they speak somewhere between announcements and the sermon. I assumed that's how it would be at her church as well. Well, you know what happens when you assume.

Unbeknownst to me, I was the only speaker for the service. I had to give the sermon. Oh my, that changed some things. I was not prepared to be the main attraction, the only attraction. I had never given a sermon in front of a congregation. Yikes! I had a lot of preparation to do. I called my friend to find out how much time I would have to speak so that I could prepare accordingly.

She said, "You can take as much time as you need."

A few days before my sermon, my friend called me and asked, "How would you like me to introduce you to the congregation? Who are you, Andrea?"

I started giving her the conventional answer that fit for the occasion, "I am a breast cancer survivor. Single. No children. I am an engineer by degree and work for XYZ. Mother of a dog named Gigi." I wasn't exactly sure what she wanted me to say. However, I could've saved both of us some time and just responded I am...*a child of God.* Emphatically, I am a child of God!!! That sums it up. I am a surrendered vessel created in His image for His use. I'm very grateful to be that and it is not something I take lightly or for granted. He chose me and I'm part of his royal priesthood. 1 Peter 2:9 (KJV) says "But ye are a chosen generation, a royal priesthood, an holy nation, a peculiar people; that ye should shew forth the praises of him who hath called you out of darkness into his marvelous light." That is good stuff. As children of God, we have royal blood flowing through our veins. We are all kings and queens.

"I AM...two of the most powerful words; what you put after them shapes your reality." This quote reminds me of something I heard Pastor Joel Osteen say. To paraphrase, he said whatever follows the words I AM, is going to come looking for you. If you say I AM BROKE, guess what, you'll be broke. If you say I AM A NOBODY, you'll be a nobody. If you say I AM "anything", you are inviting that "anything" into your life. Therefore, when I say "I AM BEAU-TIFUL," I'm inviting beauty into my life. So when I say "I AM A CHILD OF GOD," I'm inviting God into my life.

TUESDAY, NOVEMBER 22, 2011 7:49 AM; 117 days since my 2ⁿᵈ cancer diagnosis.

I. AM. TIRED!!! As I sit here doing my first brachytherapy treatment, I realize I am just tired of this. Please keep me in your prayers as I press forward.

[a very quick reflection]

I have to laugh at myself with this post. I know exactly what I just said about "I AM." I am being careful with the words I put after them, but this is my reality. I really am tired. Can this just be over? Don't judge me.

WEDNESDAY, DECEMBER 7, 2011 1:16 PM; 132 days since my 2ⁿᵈ diagnosis.

Hey there family and friends. I just wanted to let you know I have completed my last radiation treatment yesterday. Whoo Hoo. I tell you, this road has been challenging, but I am thankful that I can still praise God through all of this. "In all of this confusion/mess, there is a gift to be found." I just wanted to thank you all for your thoughts and prayers during this time. I am so appreciative. Right now, I am on break. I have a few weeks to recover and get my energy back before I start with the chemotherapy treatments. I'm not exactly sure when it will start, but I know it won't be before January 6th, which is the date of my appointment with my GYN oncologist. So I'm planning to enjoy this holiday season, rest, and continue being grateful for life. I love you all and I wish you all the best during the holiday season. Merry Christmas and have a great New Year!

[personal reflection]

There was still much more to this journey, but I didn't feel it was necessary to share my experience with the chemotherapy treatments again. This process was pretty similar to the previous one. I did have a few different side effects, but there's no need to complain. I have life!

As you may recall, during the first time around with cancer, I never questioned God. I never asked, "Why me?" However, I would be telling a fib if I said I didn't question why the second time. Maybe I wasn't moving fast enough toward my destiny of fulfilling my purpose. Maybe there were still some lessons to be learned from my experiences. Maybe it wasn't necessarily for me. I don't know. Having gone through these two battles, what I do know for sure is that I must continue to trust in the Most High God. In all things, I will put Him first. He said He will never leave me, nor forsake me until the end of the ages.

We are all stars in our own movie. As much as I would've loved not to have participated in this particular show, I couldn't just walk away because I was playing the leading role. I was the star and I had to put on my best performance and beat this cancer thing again. I AM...a conqueror!

Reflection Questions

1. *Who are you and what is the descriptor that you would put after "I AM...?"*
2. *Do others see you that way, too?*

3. *If not, how can you change their perception of you?*

19

ready. set. live...on purpose!

"LIFE HAS NO MEANING. EACH OF US HAS MEANING
AND WE BRING IT TO LIFE. IT IS A WASTE TO BE
ASKING THE QUESTION WHEN YOU ARE THE
ANSWER."

– JOSEPH CAMPBELL

One Sunday morning, I was watching Super Soul
Sunday on the Oprah Winfrey Network. Mark Nepo

was Oprah's guest for the day. Mark Nepo is a cancer survivor and also a New York Times #1 bestseller author, poet and philosopher. Toward the end of the television program, Oprah asked him what is the purpose of the human experience. His response blew me away.

Paraphrasing, he said the purpose of the human experience is for the soul to blossom in human form here on earth. Rather than finding heaven on earth, we are to release heaven by living on earth. That was an ah-ha moment for me. We are responsible for releasing heaven while on earth. Basically he was saying that while we're living on earth, we are to give of ourselves to make life better for someone else. Of course, that got me to thinking, *What is my purpose? How can I best release heaven by living on this earth?*

Trying to find my purpose isn't a new endeavor for me. It's something I've searched for quite some time. I remember once I was flying home, gazing out the window, thinking about how amazing God is. He is the creator of all things. He created the heavens and earth. The sun and the moon. He named all the stars I was observing out the cloudy window pane. He created everything...even the mosquitos. Even the skunks. Even the raccoons. Even the...well, you get the point. All the things we love and even those things we don't, He created with a purpose in mind.

I remember being asked the question, "What is the meaning of life?" It is a difficult question to answer. Joseph Campbell, an American writer said, "Life has no meaning. Each of us has meaning and we bring it to life. It is a waste to be asking the question when you are the answer." Instead of asking the "rhetorical" question, "What's the meaning of life?" I ask myself, "What gives life meaning?" The only answer I can come up with is *purpose*.

In the book, *The Purpose Driven Life*, by Rick Warren, the first sentence starts with the words "It's not about you." Wow. How is *my* purpose not about me? It's *my* purpose. The author, Rick Warren, goes on to say that the purpose of our life is far greater than our own personal fulfillment, peace of mind or even happiness. We were created for a grander purpose. A purpose that entails how we can best serve others.

The discovery of purpose is one that eludes many of us. Many can't seem to figure it out. Some go through life aimlessly. Instead of truly living, they just exist. If we put our focus on others rather than ourselves, maybe our lives would be richer. Remember, our purpose isn't about us. It's about how to best give ourselves away to others.

I continuously ask myself, "What's my purpose?"

It is my heart's desire to live in alignment with what God has purposed me to do. The Bible says in Colossians, "For in him all things were created: things in heaven and on earth, visible and invisible, whether thrones or powers or rulers or authorities; all things have been created through him and for him." I believe my purpose is to open hearts, blossom compassion, and inspire others to live their best lives through my words, whether spoken or written. That is what has led me to writing this book. My life, my cancer experiences, they aren't just for me. They are for anyone whom I'm able to touch.

All of us were created for a purpose. We all have stories that we can share. We all can be impactful. Joel Osteen once said, "As long as you have breath, someone needs your talents. Your talent is God's gift to you. What you choose to do with that talent is your gift back to Him."

When I first heard it, I paused for a moment to think about my talents and how could I share them with the world. I want to positively impact people's lives, those I know and even those who I don't. I want to challenge them to live the life they desire, the life they deserve.

I know there's a perfect plan for my life and I'm excited to see what the future holds. While I can't predict the future, I know life's too short to just let it happen. I have to make it happen. I will make the most of each moment because I don't know when it'll be over for me...*here on earth*. I'm still here for a reason.

I am not my disease, but this dis-ease, this uncomfortableness has allowed me to have a message to share. My public service announcement. I am not cancer, but it is part of my life and has given me responsibility and purpose. Friedrich Nietzsche wrote, "He who has a **why** to live for can bear almost any **how**." I receive that. As I mentioned before, I am appreciative for the platform that God has afforded me and for the opportunity to share my story. If I can just encourage people to hold on and trust God through the good and the bad, and also encourage them to get to know their breasts and check them regularly, this book will not be in vain. I just want to help save a life or a soul.

I would be remiss if I shared my experiences with you without asking you to be a partner in this journey to purpose...just for a moment. Ask yourselves, "What is my purpose? How am I giving of myself to serve others? How am I sharing my talents, experiences, skills, time, and/or money to help promote the well-being others?"

We can change the world together if we align our walk with God's purpose. You are necessary. I am necessary. We all are necessary. Somebody, some-where can benefit from what we have to offer. Live in your purpose...*on purpose.*

I believe as you continue to grow and be stretched, your purpose will transcend you to your next responsibility.

———

Reflection Questions

1. *What is your why? What's the purpose of your life?*
2. *How will you serve others?*
3. *How can you release heaven by living here on earth?*

20

live out loud (lol)

"WHEN YOU'RE FINISHED CHANGING, YOU'RE
FINISHED."

— BENJAMIN FRANKLIN

Cancer has been a great teacher. I knew I was a
strong person, but I just didn't know how strong.
I have faced death twice, overcame it both times,
and thrived afterward. I believe that is what's called
being resilient. Yes, that's me! Resilient. Sometimes,
I'm still amazed as to how well I handled the situa-

tion. This is the life I was given and I was prepared to fight with all my might. It all worked for my good.

"But as for you, ye thought evil against me; but God meant it unto good, to bring to pass, as it is this day, to save much people alive." – Genesis 50:20 (KJV)

I loved the person I was at 39 years old B.C. (Before Cancer). However, I can truly say I also admire and respect the woman I am today. I have taken life by the horns and have been riding this adventure on my terms. I live my life in color instead of black and white with shades of grey. It has been amazing! Facing death has been a conscious reminder for me to live...to live intentionally. I have to be grateful for every moment that God gives me. One day, I sat down and wrote twenty-seven experiences that I want to have before I die. I didn't want to put just anything on the list. I wanted the list to be thoughtful and challenging. One of the experiences was to meet the President of the United States of America. I didn't know how I was going to make that happen, but I knew I had to try to figure out a way.

Previously, I had read an article recently on how to cross things off of your bucket list. I don't remember everything the article said to do, but I do remember it said that in order cross some things off, you need to be ballsy. Also, it said that you need to be bold and courageous.

It just so happened that President Obama was campaigning for his 2012 bid and he was coming to town. Since I had volunteered for his campaign, I was able to get a ticket to see him. I knew in order for me to meet him, I needed to be where he was.

I was so excited that day! I left home early so I could get a good seat at the park where he was speaking. I drove thirty minutes to the event before I realized I left my ticket at home. In my excitement, I had taken the ticket out of my car so that I could take a picture of it for memories' sake. Unfortunately, I left it on my kitchen table. I rushed home during rush hour traffic, picked up the ticket, and then rushed back in order to make it there before the President's motorcade. I did not want to miss out on the opportunity to see the President. I couldn't believe how careless I was in this situation. *How could I leave the ticket at home?* Fortunately, by the time I arrived, the President hadn't. I was still able to get into the park. The bad thing was now I would have to stand because all the seats were taken. I walked around the park trying to find the best place to stand. I sneaked into the VIP area and stood in front of a tree. It was a great location because I was able to lean on the tree for support and I was only about thirty to forty feet away from where the President would speak. As I began to take pictures with my iPad, I dropped my used ticket to an Oprah Winfrey show. I had gone to see her a few months prior. That had been a dream of mine as well. As I picked up the ticket off of the ground, I began to think, *"Is this a sign?"* I realized 'Dreams Do Come True', and if I made it to the Oprah show, I can try to figure out how to meet the President.

"Be ballsy. Be bold. Be courageous." At that point, I realized that even though I had a great spot, it wasn't good enough to meet the President. I needed to move toward the front. *How am I going to do that?* Well, I decided to walk toward the front of the VIP area, and act as though I belonged there. No one said anything to me nor did they complain when I sat on the ground right in front of them, especially since it was hot outside and I had a fan.

I began fanning those around me so they would want/need me there. The President came out and spoke to the crowd for about forty-five minutes. I was able to take some great photos. After he said, "God bless you and God Bless the United States of America," I jumped to my feet. Now, I needed to figure out how I was going to get him to come my way. I needed to meet him.

I was preparing different conversation starters in

my mind that I could use to make him come my way. I mean, his speech was about healthcare reform and I just happened to be going through cancer, which is a pre-existing condition. Yes, that's it. He would *have* to come over if he saw my bald head. Fortunately, it didn't have to come to that. Thank goodness because I really didn't want to display my bald head in public. The President began greeting the people who were in the front row. Guess who was in the front row? Yes, Andrea, the girl with the fan. All of a sudden I became one of those people who was star struck. LOL.

As he was getting closer to me, I became nervous. *Is this really about to happen?* He almost rendered me speechless as he came by and shook my hand. I thanked him for what he's doing for the country and his plans with healthcare. A-M-A-Z-I-N-G!!!

I don't want you to get all caught up in my excitement. The point that I want to make about this experience is that I was able to cross it off of my list in just three weeks of writing it by being ballsy and intentional. This was a great reminder that if I want something to happen, then I have to make it happen. Do it with intentionality.

There was also a more recent experience I was able to cross off the list. I mentioned I had attended an Oprah show a few months prior to meeting the President, but that wasn't enough for me. Yes, it was great to be in her presence and in the audience with like-minded individuals, however I needed more. I wanted to touch her, talk to her, and tell her what she means to me. I know there are many fans out there who feel the same way I do since she is such a powerful woman.

Oprah was doing "The Life You Want" tour which was a weekend workshop with herself and some of her top thought leaders. Once again, I knew if I wanted to meet Oprah, I needed to be where she was. Instead of just attending the workshop, I chose to participate in the VIP experience. Being a VIP allowed me the opportunity to take a picture with Oprah. How exciting was that going to be?!? I needed to figure out what I wanted to say to her when we took our picture together.

After carefully preparing the thoughts I wanted to share with her, she stood in front of the audience and mentioned she didn't want to hear our life stories when she took pictures with us. She said that she understood we all had a story to tell, but she didn't have all night to listen to them. Dangit!

Oh well, I guessed it would be enough to just meet her and take a picture. As it was approaching my turn, I began to think, how can I be ballsy in this situation. I could not let this opportunity pass me by without attempting to have the conversation I wanted to have with Oprah. As I approached Oprah like a little school girl, she did something totally unexpected. She rubbed my hair. *Who does that?* Oprah...and thank goodness she did because that opened the door for me to have the conversation I wanted to have. She told me she loved my haircut.

"Thanks Oprah. I love you!" I shared with her how she had inspired me to live my best life. I told her about my battles with cancer and how I would watch the Oprah Winfrey Network as I sat home through surgeries, chemotherapy and radiation. We hugged, we laughed, we gave each other high-five. She told me the world needed to hear my story and that she couldn't wait until I shared it.

How amazing is that! How amazing is she! My photo even turned out to be amazing! You would've thought that we had been friends forever. Honestly, I can say that experience was life changing for me. Besides Oprah being who she is, I learned a lesson. You have to be willing to seize the moment and not let the opportunity pass you by. I could've just let Oprah rub my hair, then stood next to her and took the picture, but that experience wouldn't have been as amazing as the one I created...with her help, of course. I came back home so energized, so ready to live my best life, so ready to live the life of my dreams.

I want to remind you that dreams do come true, no matter how big or small. You just have to be willing to take the risk associated with helping to realize them. I say to you, "Dream BIG! Dream the impossible." It is only impossible until someone does it. "You may never know what results come from your action. But if you do nothing, there will be no results." – Ghandi

I mentioned there were twenty-seven experiences on my list. Some I have crossed off at this point, and some I haven't. One of my biggest desires would be to meet at least one of the children I sponsor in Africa or South America. Will it happen? *I'm not sure.* But I can continue to try to figure it out a way to make it happen. As you can see, I didn't choose easy, doable experiences. I chose ones that would require some ingenuity to achieve. Now do I think I'll achieve them all? *I don't know.* However, I know I'll enjoy the journey as I attempt to complete them.

Reflection Questions

1. *What are five things you would love to experience in your lifetime?*

2. *How can you be more ballsy, more courageous, and bolder to ensure you have these desired experiences?*

21

dare to do you

> "THOSE WHO DARE TO FAIL MISERABLY CAN ACHIEVE
> GREATLY."
>
> – JOHN F. KENNEDY

───────

When I chose the title of this chapter, I did it intentionally. "Dare To Do You" requires you to take action and live an authentic, unapologetic, highest version of self. I want to challenge you to take action now and live the life you desire. You deserve it. I've shared my story and you can see how my life has changed...mostly for the better. I would love for you to do some introspective reflection of who you are and who you want to become.

The word "dare" requires you to have courage. According to <u>dictionary.com</u>, courage is defined as the quality of mind or spirit that enables a person to face difficulty, danger, pain, etc., without fear. In other words, it's feeling the fear and doing it anyway.

"Have I not commanded you? Be strong and coura-geous. Do not be terrified; do not be discouraged, for the Lord your God will be with you wherever you go." –
Joshua 1:9 (NIV)

I am challenging you to take a look within your-self and courageously step out on faith and do YOU. Dare to live the best version of yourself. Jonas Salk said, "Hope lies in dreams, in imagination, and in the courage of those who dare to make dreams into real-ity." Live the life you dream about. Remember, God is with you.

The late Dr. Myles Monroe, a Christian minister, once said, "The poorest person in the world is one without a dream." Ask yourself, "Do you want to be poor? Or do you want to be rich, rich in the possibil-ities?" For me, the answer is simple. I want to be rich in the possibilities. I will live my life continuing to dream bigger dreams and striving to make an impact in this world.

I believe we have to be more intentional, more deliberate in our actions as we strive to live our best lives. We have to dream big and trust that any anything dreamt is one that can be fulfilled. Phil Rozenzweig stated, "The failure to act is a greater sin than taking action and failing, because action brings at least a possibility of success, whereas inaction brings none."

Wait a minute, why am I talking about *we* all of a sudden? We know this book is mainly about me, so I will stop focusing on the *we* and focus on the...wait for it, "I." I know you may have thought I was going to say "me," but that would've been too much like right. Okay, that was a little corny, but I needed a segue back to me...*just for a moment.* I wanted to share what I've been doing since my victory over cancer.

For the first time ever, I developed a mantra for my life. It's a work in progress, meaning it may evolve into something else at some point, but right now my mantra is, *"My playing small does not serve the world. Think BIG. Dream BIG. EXPECT THE GREAT!"*

The inspiration for this came from Marianne Williamson's book, *A Return to Love.* In her book, she wrote, "Your playing small does not serve the world. There is nothing enlightened about shrinking so that other people won't feel insecure around you." This statement resonated with me. It caused me to pause and think about my life and ask the question, "Why I am playing small?" Nelson Mandela said it another way, "There is no passion to be found in playing small – in settling for a life that's less than the one you are capable of living." By living a life less than the one I should, I am settling. In essence, I'm insulting God by playing small and playing safe. I must play big. I must strive to make a difference in this world, strive to be the difference.

I am courageously stepping out on faith, playing big, dreaming the impossible, and trusting God for the extraordinary. I will no longer put any limits on what He will do in my life and what He will reveal.

I must admit, after my first battle against cancer, I became fearless. The things I wouldn't do before, now I can't wait to do them. Skydiving, *no biggie*. Flying lessons, *no biggie*. Scuba diving, *no biggie*. Okay, so I've already gone skydiving and taken flying lessons, but I hadn't gone scuba diving yet. One day.

My experiences taught me I couldn't have faith and fear. I couldn't have one arm latched on to fear, while the other was latched on to faith. That would leave me paralyzed and unable to move forward. If I totally put my trust in God, I couldn't be scared of the journey I had to take.

I am sharing these words with you about fear because it shouldn't have a place in your heart. I know we are spiritual beings having a natural experience, but we still have a human nature. It is human to be afraid of something, but during that time, we have to lean on God, trust Him, and tap into our spiritual selves.

After going through both cancer journeys, I started to think about the things I wanted to accomplish during my lifetime. I have launched my coaching, training and speaking business, Andrea Campbell, LLC. I want to help people live their best lives...the lives they deserve. I provide my clients tools that will help them in their personal transformation. They will be able to clarify their purpose and vision, to strategize and plan, and to change their mindset so they will succeed at higher levels. I am excited about helping people transform their perspective, discover their identity, and explore the possibilities. If you would like more information, you can find more information on my website AndreaDCampbell.com.

I've also become an inspirational speaker, which you can also call an inspiring motivational speaker. I've found myself having more opportunities to speak and share my cancer journey. I share the experiences, lessons learned and my resiliency with any-one who will listen.

You may ask, "How far will I go with this?" My answer is that I'm not sure yet. I am openly allowing God to use me. I can't wait to see where He takes me. He can dream a bigger dream than I can even imagine for myself.

To paraphrase another quote by Dr. Myles Monroe, he said the wealthiest place on earth is the cemetery. There lies the greatest treasure of untapped potential and unrealized dreams. I don't want to leave this earthly life being *full* of unrealized dreams and unused talents. I want to leave here on *empty*. I want to realize my full potential and use it for good.

Not too long ago, I was at a professional conference in Atlanta. I met up with a former executive at my company. I needed some advice about my career and the direction it was heading. This is someone whom I hold in high regard. She is an amazing individual and I can't wait until she decides to write her book. Her story is remarkable, powerful, and truly impactful.

Even though she was preparing to head to the airport to travel back home, she carved out forty-five minutes to meet me for coffee. I was so appreciative for that because I really wanted to pick her brain and get some clarity.

Somehow our conversation turned away from my job and led to my personal life. She began coaching me on the spot. She asked questions that forced me to do some deeper soul-searching. She told me that my purpose was being held hostage. She challenged me to release it and to be bold as I walk in it. Wow. That was intense. I didn't realize I was in my own way of walking in my purpose. Also, at some point, she told me that she sees me on a big stage. Wow again. I hadn't had that vision for myself yet.

We also talked about the giraffe and turtle analogy that I mentioned earlier in the book. She told me that because I am a giraffe, I can't survive trying to be on the same level of the turtles. She was right. God has given me the vision of a giraffe and not the turtle.

After our conversation, she asked if she could pray for me. Did I mention she's an ordained minister, too? She prayed that I'd have clarity in my path as I walked in my purpose. By the time the prayer was over, we were both crying. One other thing she prayed was for God to give me an unimaginable sign within a week so I would know I was on the right path. Now, I know God is capable of doing whatever

He wants, but I had no idea what this sign was going to be or if I would even recognize it.

I tell you, it wasn't but three days later my sign appeared. A college friend sent me a picture she had taken off of her TV. It was a picture of me plastered on the screen behind Oprah on her Life Class show. I had to laugh. One, because I had seen that particular episode a couple of times and never did I see my photo in the background. Secondly, because I don't even know how my picture got there. I'm sure I had sent it at some point, but I don't remember.

I knew that was my sign. That prayer was being answered. God showed me something unimaginable by being there on stage with Oprah. Now, I know it may not have been my stage, but I was on a stage of sorts...with Oprah, of all people. Sometimes it helps for people to share their vision of you that may be bigger than the one you can see for yourself. I can't wait to see what's in store for me.

Instead of just growing older, I will continue to grow bolder. I will trust that God will continue to show me the unimaginable while dwelling in the possibilities.

I would love to start a non-profit organization focusing on women going through cancer. The thought first came to mind after I was diagnosed with breast cancer. At that point, I wanted to specifically help women who were going through breast cancer or had gone through it previously. However, after the uterine cancer diagnosis, I thought maybe my scope had been too narrow. Instead of just dealing with women who were affected by breast cancer, I desire to focus on women who have battled any type of cancer.

In preparation, I'm learning about the ins and outs of running a non-profit by serving on the board of an organization which supports women who are currently undergoing breast cancer treatment with emergency financial assistance. Even though I'm not at a place to start my non-profit, I know I need to give back and use my talents and experiences to help others. "Never respect men merely for their riches, but rather for their philanthropy; we do not value the sun for its height, but for its use." – Gamaliel Bailey. God didn't create us to just sit pretty, He wants us to use our gifts to help others.

Years ago, I heard Les Brown speak during a conference. If you aren't familiar with him, he is a dynamic motivational speaker who also happens to be a two-time cancer survivor. During his speech, he said that love is like perfume. You can't spray it on someone else without getting some on yourself. This analogy also applies when you give of yourself, you will reap the rewards just as the person you are giving it to. Be mindful of that and figure out a way to give to someone else.

If you're having difficulties thinking about whose life you can improve, find an organization or align with a cause that you're passionate about. If you can't find one you're interested in, helping with cancer patients and research is an option because cancer will unfortunately touch us all in some way...at some point in our lives.

Here are a few statistics from the American Cancer Society. In 2015, there will be an estimated 1,658,370 new cancer cases diagnosed. There will be 589,430 cancer deaths in the U.S. That's about 1,620 people per day. Cancer remains the second most common cause of death in the U.S., accounting for nearly 1 of every 4 deaths. Data shows 1 in 2 males will develop cancer compared to 1 in 3 females.

As you can see, cancer is prevalent in our society. Because of this, it is important to find a cure, determine the causes through research, and most importantly help those in need who are battling the disease.

Five years ago, before being diagnosed, I couldn't have imagined my passion to be around helping those who have gone through cancer. It's something how life goes sometimes.

I treasure this thing called life. I can't settle for just existing when I know that living is available to me. I will make my life count and live each moment as if there may not be another one. Nothing in life is guaranteed. Tomorrow is not guaranteed. Our next breath is not guaranteed. But as long as we have breath, we should make our lives count.

Reflection Questions

1. *What actions will you take to live an authentic, unapologetic, higher version of yourself?*
2. *How daring will you be?*

22

on to the next...

"WHEN A THING IS DONE, IT'S DONE. DON'T LOOK
BACK. LOOK FORWARD TO YOUR NEXT OBJECTIVE."

— GEORGE C. MARSHALL

———

The person I was on October 8, 2009 is no longer.
The old Andrea had to die. I needed my old habits,
thoughts, behavior to die so that I could transform
into the person I am today. Even still, I don't believe
that this experience was just for me. I believe I went
through this experience so I can help others through

their difficulties. My testimony is to give hope to those who are hopeless, strength to those who are weak, inspiration to those who need inspiring, and empower to those who need to be empowered.

Luke 22:31-32 says, "Simon, Simon, Satan has asked to sift all of you as wheat. But I have prayed for you, Simon, that your faith may not fail. And when you have turned back, strengthen your brothers." Thank you Jesus. *It's not just about me.* I am to use what I've learned to help my fellow brothers (and sisters). I respect and acknowledge that I am a spiritual being just having a human experience. I pray I don't lose what I've learned spiritually through this transformation. My faith has never been tested as much as it had been going through this adversity. But I know His grace and mercy is sufficient. I will continue to follow Him as He orders my steps toward my purpose.

A couple of years ago, I remember having a conversation with a friend of mine, who happens to be an atheist. He asked me, "How can you believe in a god that would allow something this bad happen to you? Is that how he treats good people?"

I told him, "Everything that I go through is for my good. I believe that. But you're missing the main point. Whether I continue to live here on earth, or go on to glory, I win. The devil will be defeated and I still win." I believe the promises God has given me.

Honestly, I did not know how my cancer battles would end. Regardless of the outcome, God would be glorified.

As I'm sitting here writing this book, I just heard that Stuart Scott, a sportscaster from ESPN, passed away from a long battle with cancer. Even though he lost his battle, he gave the world a profound way to look at his fight when he was honored at the 2014 ESPY awards show. During his speech, he said, "When you die, it does not mean that you lose to cancer. You beat cancer by how you live, why you live, and in the manner in which you live." I will continue to beat cancer by *how I live*, discovering the *why I live*, and in the *manner that I live*. I live to glorify God and to give Him praises for who He is and all He continues to do in my life.

Like many others, I am saddened by the passing of Stuart Scott who was as cool as the other side of the pillow. He was entertaining to watch on TV. However, I have a little guilt about his passing. They call it survivor's guilt. I know it sounds crazy, but when I hear of others who have succumbed to this deadly disease, I can't help to think why did they die and I get to live. I have to remind myself that it's simply not my time. God is still using me and for that, I am grateful.

It's been six years since my first cancer diagnosis and I am finally sharing my story for the world to read. I always felt that my story would be told, but evidently my timing was different than God's timing. God revealed to me that there was a reason I needed to delay writing my story. I was still living it. Now I'm finally able to share with you.

Even though, I still am dealing with the effects of the cancer treatments, I continue to praise Him. Through it all, He still deserves the praise. There were times when I felt as though I was taking God for granted, but what I realized is that I wasn't taking Him for granted, I was just confident in His capabilities and what He could do in my life. I knew He was the Ultimate Healer and He has the ability to perform a miracle and cure me. Because He did, I am thankful. I will continually praise Him because I know things could've turned out much worse. But God...

God has been so good to me through it all. Is my life perfect? *Of course not.* Am I cancer-free? *Yes.* Do I still have other residual side effects? *Yes.* Do I still have joint pain in my fingers? *Daily, and it causes me difficulties when trying to do normal day-to-day activities.*

Do my feet swell and cause me pain? *Unfortunately, yes.*

This battle was not easy but I made it through. Even with the scars, the constant pains, and chemo brain, I made it through. Some things I'll never understand, but I just have to accept. I've learned to not sweat the small stuff. Instead of focusing on what's bad, I've chosen to focus on the good. I count my blessings every day. I've become more diligent in practicing the art of gratitude. It is amazing how this practice has shifted my mindset. Instead of focusing on lack and scarcity, I choose to focus on the abundance in my life.

Gratitude takes away fear; it is difficult to be grateful and afraid at the same time. I heard one of Oprah's thought leaders state that gratitude is the state of BE-ing (intentional thought) and not a state of DO-ing (thinking something has to be done). If we deliberately choose to be grateful, we can "Unlock the fullness of life. It turns what we have into enough and more. It turns denial into acceptance, chaos to order, confusion to clarity. It can turn a meal into a feast, a house into a home, a stranger into a friend." – Melody Beattie.

Life after cancer isn't easy. Currently, I'm still taking my chemo medication daily which causes me a lot of pain. Initially, I was only supposed to take this drug for five years, but my oncologist suggested that I consider taking the drug for an additional five years. I guess there's some new research data that has shown an increase in survivability if the meds are taken for ten-year period. Since I was considered *young* when I was diagnosed with the breast cancer, my oncologist thought it would be best for me to continue on the medication if I want to live a long life. As you can imagine, I wasn't happy to hear this. I was tired of being in pain. I had even planned on having a celebration once I had finished taking the medication. Unfortunately, that celebration won't take place for another five years.

There are still moments when I get nervous about a recurrence of cancer. If I have an out-of-the-ordinary ache or pain, I get nervous. Even if my pinky finger hurts, I get nervous. When I have my routine follow-ups, I get nervous. When I have scans performed, I get nervous. I can't let my nervousness cause me to worry. I have to continuously remind myself to trust God and know He is still in control.

As I begin planning for the next chapter of my life, I'm reflecting on all the blessings that have been bestowed upon me. You are included in those blessings. You took the time to go on this beautiful journey with me. Thank you. My intentions in sharing my story were to inform, inspire, and serve as a reminder to live...courageously, intentionally and purposefully. "Inspiration does not favor those that sit still...it dances with the daring." – Unknown.

As you experience trials and tribulations in your life, whether it happens to be cancer, some other ailment, or even a stronghold that has you bound, remember not to give up. Be bold. Be daring. Be resilient. Remember that in spite of your situation, the common thread for victory is having faith in God. The Son continues to shine even through the darkest storms.

I am looking forward to receiving all that God has for me. I know my latter will be much greater. Prior to cancer, I considered my life to be pretty good. I was looking good, feeling good, and living good. I had the things that people grow up dreaming about: my own home, nice car, decent money, and a career. However, good was not enough. I was not created just to have a good life. I was created to have a better than good life. A meaningful life. A life of significance, where I know my life matters and I'm living in my purpose.

Reflection Questions

1. *What lessons will you take from the past and how will you use them moving forward?*
2. *What actions will you take today to change your tomorrow?*

Afterword

Now, I understand why people say writing a book is like going through a pregnancy. Instead of nine months, I had this book in my belly for almost five years. However, after all the ups, downs, complications, and pains, I have now given birth to my baby, *The Beautiful Journey*. I am teary-eyed as I write this. I can't believe this dream has finally come to fruition. It is a dream fulfilled. Had someone told me ten years ago that I would be an author, I would have thought that person was crazy. I wasn't even the biggest fan of writing at that time. It wasn't even a dream I had dreamt at that point in my life.

It wasn't until I began blogging during my journey that the idea was put into my head. I remember reading through the comments of those who were following my blogs, and "Cookie Lady" mentioned that I should write a book. My first thought was "*No way.*" I am very private when it comes to the most intimate parts of my life. I don't willingly share those details with just anyone. Anyway, who would want to read my story, or any story about cancer for that matter? Heck, I wasn't even sure I wanted to have to relive that period of my life again. However, I was reminded that my story isn't one about cancer per se, but how I claimed victory over it.

Thank you Cookie Lady for planting the seed.

Cookie Lady's real identity will remain anonymous, but I have to share how she got her nickname. Every time I hear this story, I laugh so hard.

Some years ago, one of my friends started working at a new job. After a few months into her role as a manager, she already had established a pretty good relationship with one of her employees, Cookie Lady. While conversing with my friend, Cookie Lady mentioned how she was forced to interview for the same manager position as my friend. Cookie Lady didn't want the job and hadn't interviewed in over twenty-five years. Cookie Lady proceeded to tell my friend a story about her experience.

At the time of her interview, Cookie Lady was on disability due to an issue with her back. She was in so much pain that her husband had to help her get dressed and into the car so that she could make it to the interview. She had taken a Percocet earlier that morning to help with her back pain caused by sitting.

Needless to say, she was a little 'under the influence' when she arrived for the interview. Once she entered the interviewing room, she was greeted by seven interviewers: the Director of Finance, the Deputy Director of Finance, the Director of Operations, the Deputy Director of Operations, the Director of Engineering and Construction, an engineer, and a consultant. Besides the seven interviewers being in the room, there were also some cookies sitting on a table in the corner.

Before the interview began, Cookie Lady whispered to the Director of Finance, "I can't believe you're making me do this." The Director of Finance and the others proceeded with the interview. She was doing a pretty good job of answering the questions, that is until they asked one about the budget. She wasn't sure how to answer the question so she decided to take another approach.

She said, "You know what, instead of trying to answer that question since I don't know how, why don't we all have a cookie instead?"

What? Who does that in an interview? That is hilarious to me. After that remark, they all enjoyed a cookie and the interview ended.

When my friend called me to tell me the story, we laughed so hard. Tears were flowing. I had to go down to their job to meet Cookie Lady and see who had offered (and eaten) cookies during an interview.

Even now, I am laughing as I type this. Needless to say, from that day on, she has been known to me and my friend as Cookie Lady. I didn't know her real name for years. Anyway, I just wanted to share this funny story with you. Thanks, Cookie Lady, for the laughter...and for getting me to think about becoming an author.

I am appreciative for everyone who has pushed me through this process. This book has been a long time coming but I'm glad I'm able to finally share it with you. I hope you enjoyed reading about my beautiful journey and can now appreciate why I opened the book with the phrase *"Everybody should have to have cancer!"* Trust me, I don't wish this illness on anyone, but I would love for everyone to experience all the lessons and blessings that were because of it. There were a lot of ups and downs, good times and bad, but still, in this mess there were blessings to be found. I've learned that love is the only way to win over adversity and God is Love.

I will leave you with my grandmother's favorite scripture, Psalm 23. I know I've already shared it in the book, but it has special memories. As a child, this was the first Bible chapter I memorized. As I matured in my relationship with God, I now have a better understanding of the words in this psalm. I realize that the first verse is pretty much all that's needed to know to get through life's adversities, which we will all face.

The Lord is my Shepherd; I shall not want. Knowing that I shall not want for anything is enough.

Psalm 23 (KJV)

[1] *The Lord is my Shepherd; I shall not want.* [2] *He maketh me to lie down in green pastures: he leadeth me beside the still waters.* [3] *He restoreth my soul: he leadeth me in the paths of righteousness for His name's sake.* [4] *Yea, though I walk through the valley of the shadow of death, I will fear no evil: for thou art with me; thy rod and thy staff, they comfort me.* [5] *Thou preparest a table before me in the presence of mine enemies; thou anointest my head with oil; my cup runneth over.* [6] *Surely goodness and mercy shall follow me all the days of my life: and I will dwell in the House of the Lord forever.* AMEN.

Standing on God's Promises

Although this adventure hadn't been easy, I am grateful for the word of God. In His book, He had given me many promises to stand on throughout this beautiful journey. I've already shared some of God's promises throughout the book, but I would love to share with you some of my other favorite ones.

"For God so loved the world that He gave His one and only Son, that whoever believes in him shall not perish but have eternal life."
John 3:16 (NIV)

"Ask and it will be given to you; seek and you will find; knock and the door will be opened to you. For everyone who ask receives; the one who seeks finds; and to the one who knocks, the door will be opened."
Matthew 7:7-8 (NIV)

*"The Lord is good, a refuge in times of trouble. He cares
for those who trust in Him."*
Nahum 1:7 (NIV)

"I will never leave thee, nor forsake thee."
Hebrews 13:5 (NIV)

*"Take delight in the Lord, and he will give you the desires
of your heart. Commit your way to the Lord; trust in him
and he will do this."*
Psalm 37:4-5 (NIV)

*"For I am the Lord, your God, who takes hold of your
right hand and says to you, Do not fear; I will help you."*
Isaiah 41:13 (NIV)

"No weapon formed against me shall prosper."
Isaiah 54:17a (NIV)

*"For I know the plans I have for you, declares the
Lord, plans to prosper you and not to harm you, plans to
give you hope and a future."*
Jeremiah 29:11 (NIV)

*"Trust in the Lord with all your heart and lean not on
your own understanding; in all your ways submit to
him, and he will make your paths straight."*
Proverb 3:5-6 (NIV)

"And we know that all things work together for good them that love God, to them who are the called according to his purpose."
Romans 8:28 (NIV)

References

[1] Bishop Paul Morton, "Be Blessed," Songwriter: Kurt Carr, 2006

[2] Milton Brunson, "Safe in His Arms," Songwriter: Darius Brooks, 1998

[3] Thomas Ken, "Doxology," 1674. These lyrics are actually the last verse of a longer hymn, Awake, My Soul, and with the Sun.

[4] Richard Smallwood with Vision, "Center Of My Joy," Songwriters: William Gaither, Gloria Gaither, and Richard Smallwood, 2002

[5] John P. Kee, "Life and Favor," Songwriter: John P. Kee, Kee Music Group, 2012

With Gratitude and Appreciation

First and foremost, I must to give honor to God. If it wasn't for Him...I couldn't even imagine. Thank you not only for sparing my life, but for choosing me as Your child. I am so not deserving, not in the least bit, but I'm more than thankful to be a part of Your kingdom. You are the only reason that this ugly ordeal transformed into the beautiful journey it has become. Abba Father, I love you with my whole heart.

There are a few folk who I have to single out because of their participation in helping me create my personal masterpiece. First of all, I have to thank my friend, Tracy. I want you to know I really appreciate all the countless hours you listened to me as I bounced ideas off of you while I was writing this book. Also, I am grateful for the time you spent reading and editing my book. You were the first to receive my manuscript when it was a very, very

rough draft. I appreciate all of your suggestions...even the one about the raccoon.

Alvin, I am so glad we reconnected after all these
years. I appreciate you for being a catalyst in helping
me finish my book and for holding me accountable.
You reinforced my desire to touch someone's life
with my words and my journey. It's more than a mere
want – it's a responsibility. Thank you for taking the
time edit my manuscript and providing great feed-
back. You are truly special.

To my family, thank you all for the love and support you have shown me throughout my life and
especially during my cancer journey. You all
are incredible and I love you for it.

To my closest and dearest friends, you are my
chosen family. Thank you for being a part of my life.
I don't know if I should even try to start naming folk
because I will probably miss somebody. Blame it on
the chemo. There are a few that I have to acknowledge by name, though. Jackie, Leighton, Nakia, Cassandra, Nichelle, Justine, and LaTina, thanks for
your love, support and encouragement...from the
bottom of my heart.

Also, I have to give a "shout out" to some folk.
Scott, you were there encouraging me in the begin-
ning to write my book through all of our FB chats.
Brookie, you advocated for the title you suggested.

Maybe I can use it for my next book. Lori, thanks for reminding me that the enemy of good is perfect. I have come to accept that my book is imperfectly perfect.

To my sweet nephew, Elijah, you bring so much joy to my life. Continue being such an awesome kid. I wish you the best life. I love you.

To my cousin/niece/daughter, Teryn, you are such a beautiful and compassionate soul. Even though you had a difficult time watching me go through this, you continued to encourage me throughout my journey. Thank you for reminding me to "drink more water today, tomorrow, and the next day." Also, thanks for reminding me to eat when I didn't feel like it. I love the person you are...and have always been. You deserve all the blessings that come your way.

To Joshua, thank you for honoring me with your first (and hopefully only) tattoo. You are a wonderful young man. I'm proud to call you my godson. I love you.

To my lovely goddaughter, Aleena, I am so proud of the young lady you are and I wish you much success as you begin your journey at the University of Pennsylvania.

I am so blessed to have my Raggedies in my life. Aaliyah (Raggedy #1), India (Raggedy #2) and

Erin (Raggedy #3), you all are beautiful, intelligent and loving young ladies. Even though I call you my Raggedies, you are far from it. You continually make me proud. You deserve all that your heart desires.

Since my cancer journey, God saw fit to bless me with two additional godchildren. To Grayson and Sydney, I am honored to be your godmother. You're so full of life and so very smart. Remember to dream BIG.

To Dr. Bertice Berry, thank you, thank you, thank you. You are a beautiful, brilliant and amazing spirit with so much wisdom. I appreciate you and I'm grateful to have you in my life. I am honored you chose to write my foreword.

To Dannie Baker, whom I lovingly call daddy, it has been hard watching you go through dementia. Even though you are confused a lot of the time, I truly believe you know who I am when I'm there with you. Even though you may not understand these words, I have to share them with the world. I appreciate you and I'm grateful to have had you as my dad. Thank you for treating me like I was your favorite child. Without you and your DNA, Andrea wouldn't be Andrea. *"Did I just speak in third person?"* Anyway, I love you...

Since I initially express my gratitude and appreciation above, my dad has ascended to heaven. I'm keeping these words of expression in here because this is what I was feeling when I completed writing this book. I love you, daddy. Rest in peace.

Also, I would also like to thank my mommy, Jeri Campbell. You have always been a source of inspiration in my life. You are my rock. You amazed me with your strength as I went through cancer. I know it was difficult watching your only child, go through this, but I am appreciative of the fact you allowed me to draw from your strength. Throughout my life, you have been my biggest cheerleader. Thank you loving me, believing in me, molding me and even bragging on me when it would drive me crazy. I know you only did it because you were proud of me. I'm so grateful that God chose you to be my mother, my hero. Your unconditional love is unmatched. I love you to the moon, the sun, around each star, and back.

Lastly, if you're reading this, thank you. I appreciate you taking this journey with me. I wish you a lifetime of love, peace and blessings.

Hugs and Kisses...

Andrea Dyan Campbell

About Andrea

Andrea Dyan Campbell, MS, MBA is the CEO of Andrea Campbell, LLC. She is an author, inspirational speaker and trainer. After years of working in corporate America as a successful engineer, salesperson and trainer, she decided to follow her heart's desire to help others live their best lives...*on purpose.* She firmly believes you deserve to be the best you yet. She's passionate about inspiring and motivating others to make that intentional change in their lives to achieve the greatest rewards that they can be proud of.

Andrea is enjoying her life as she walks in her purpose. She currently lives in Cleveland, OH with her dog, Gigi. She has seven beautiful godchildren: Joshua, Aleena, Aaliyah, India, Erin, Grayson, and Sydney.

Find her on the web: <u>AndreaDCampbell.com</u>.